Palliative Care in Clini

Giovambattista Zeppetella

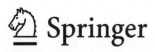 Springer

G. Zeppetella, FRCGP, FRCP
St Clare Hospice
Hastingwood
UK

ISBN 978-1-4471-2842-7   ISBN 978-1-4471-2843-4   (eBook)
DOI 10.1007/978-1-4471-2843-4
Springer Dordrecht Heidelberg New York London

Library of Congress Control Number: 2012938640

A catalogue record for this book is available from the British Library

Contents

Author Biography

Giovambattista 'John' Zeppetella, **FRCGP**, **FRCP**, graduated from University College London, UK where he obtained a degree in Physiology before qualifying in Medicine in 1985 and entered Palliative Medicine in 1987. Dr Zeppetella was appointed consultant in palliative medicine at St Joseph's Hospice in London in 1993 where he later became Deputy Medical Director and honorary consultant at St Bartholomew's and the London NHS Trust. Since July 2003, Dr Zeppetella has been Medical Director at St Clare Hospice, Hastingwood, UK and honorary consultant at the Princess Alexandra NHS Trust.

Dr Zeppetella is actively involved in education and has contributed to educational activities at the Universities of London, Bristol, Cardiff, and Cambridge. He has a number of research interests, and publications include papers on dyspnea, adherence to medication, topical administration of opioids to painful wounds, and breakthrough pain in cancer patients, and has contributed chapters to several textbooks including the *Oxford Textbook of Palliative Medicine* and is a referee for several peer-reviewed journals.

Introduction

Doctors are men who prescribe medicines of which they know little, to cure diseases of which they know less, in human beings of whom they know nothing.

Voltaire

It has always been important to me that as clinicians we should challenge Voltaire's point of view by ensuring that we gain a better understanding of therapies, illness, and people. I have been fortunate to be part of the relatively young specialty of palliative medicine and to be taught by some of the protagonists of the hospice movement who instilled within me the importance of education and training. It has always been a source of pride and satisfaction to me when colleagues in whose training I have been involved take up their own specialist post and subsequently help shape the specialty.

My original career aim was general practice, but I steered away from it after enjoying the experience of a community palliative care post at St Joseph's Hospice, London as part of my vocational training scheme. Throughout my time in the specialty, however, I have continued to be involved in community palliative care. There have been many changes over the years, and helping to care for patients in their own homes still provides me with job satisfaction, despite an increasingly complicated and often fragmented social and healthcare system that offers challenges for patients, caregivers, and healthcare professionals alike.

My intention in writing this companion guide is to provide a text for community healthcare professionals, drawing on the experience that I have been fortunate enough to gain. Clinicians in specialist training may also find it of help. The focus has primarily been on patients with cancer, and I have endeavored to provide up-to-date information, drawing on established textbooks and guidelines, wherever possible. Given the ever-increasing use of the Internet, websites are also cited. I hope that the information provided will assist clinicians in the care of their patients, in an effort to make a difficult time a little easier.

John Zeppetella, 2011

Acknowledgments

I would like to thank my friends and colleagues at St Joseph's Hospice, London and St Clare Hospice, Hastingwood for their support over the past 20 years, especially BLB, whose support, and encouragement while writing this companion guide, has been much appreciated.

Particular thanks are extended to MDR, who has been a close colleague, friend, and companion and to my wonderful daughters, Elizabeth and Claudia.

Finally, and most importantly, I give my thanks and appreciation to all the patients whom I have had the privilege to meet over the years. It is they and their loved ones who have been my teachers, instructing me what to do and, more importantly, what not to do.

Abbreviations

5HT	5-hydroxtryptamine or serotonin
ACP	Advance care planning
ACS	Anorexia/cachexia syndrome
AIDS	Acquired immune deficiency syndrome
ALA	α-lipoic acid
ANH	Artificial nutrition and hydration
APM	Association for Palliative Medicine
BPI	Brief Pain Inventory
CBC	Complete blood count
CEA	Carcinoembryonic antigen
CNS	Central nervous system
COPD	Chronic obstructive pulmonary disease
CPR	Cardiopulmonary resuscitation
CSCI	Continuous subcutaneous infusion
CT	Computed tomography
CTZ	Chemoreceptor trigger zone
DNACPR	Do-not-attempt cardiopulmonary resuscitation
DNAR	Do-not-attempt resuscitation
DSM	*Diagnostic and Statistical Manual of Mental Disorders*
DVLA	Driver and Vehicle Licensing Agency
ECOG	Eastern Co-operative Oncology Group
G-CSF	Granulocyte colony-stimulating factor
GI	Gastrointestinal
GSF	Gold Standards Framework
GP	General practitioner
HADS	Hospital Anxiety and Depression Scale
Hb	Hemoglobin
LANSS	Leeds Assessment of Neuropathic Signs and Symptoms
LCP	Liverpool Care Pathway
LFT	Liver function test
MAOI	Monoamine oxidase inhibitor
MRI	Magnetic resonance imaging
NRS	Numerical rating scale

NSAID	Non-steroidal anti-inflammatory drug
PPC	Preferred Priorities for Care
PPI	Proton pump inhibitor
SCC	Spinal cord compression
SSRI	Selective serotonin reuptake inhibitor
SVC	Superior vena cava
SVCO	Superior vena cava obstruction
SVCS	Superior vena cava syndrome
TCA	Tricyclic antidepressant
U&Es	Urea and electrolytes
VAS	Visual analog scales
WHO	World Health Organization

Prescriptions

bd	Twice daily
cap	Capsule
inj	Injection
iv	Intravenously
mixt	Mixture
od	Once daily
po	Orally
pr	Rectally
prn	As required
q3h	3 hourly
q4h	4 hourly
q6h	6 hourly
q8h	8 hourly
qds	Four times daily
sc	Subcutaneously
sl	Sublingually
stat	Immediately
supp	Suppository
tab	Tablet
tds	Three times daily

Chapter 1

Introduction to Palliative Care

Definition of Palliative Care

Palliative care (from the Latin *palliare*, "to cloak") describes any form of medical care or treatment that concentrates on reducing the severity of disease symptoms, rather than striving to halt, delay, or reverse the progression of the disease itself, or provide a cure. A number of definitions of palliative care exist in the literature, including the recent World Health Organization's statement [1] that describes:

> … an approach that improves the quality of life of patients and their families facing the problems associated with life-threatening illness, through the prevention and relief of suffering by means of early identification and impeccable assessment and treatment of pain and other problems, physical, psychosocial, and spiritual.

In essence, the goal of palliative care is to prevent and relieve suffering and to improve the quality of life for people facing serious, complex illness (Figure 1.1). To be successful, palliative care requires attention to all aspects of a patient's suffering, which requires input or assistance using a multiprofessional approach (Figure 1.2).

Principles of Palliative Care

The principles of palliative care might simply be regarded as those of good clinical practice and include the following:

G. Zeppetella, *Palliative Care in Clinical Practice*,
DOI 10.1007/978-1-4471-2843-4_1,
© Springer-Verlag London 2012

Palliative care components

- Symptom control
- Effective communication
- Rehabilitation
- Continuity of care
- Terminal care
- Support in bereavement
- Education
- Research

Figure 1.1 Palliative care components. (Data from Mount et al. [2]. Reproduced with permission from John Wiley and Sons)

A multiprofessional approach to palliative care

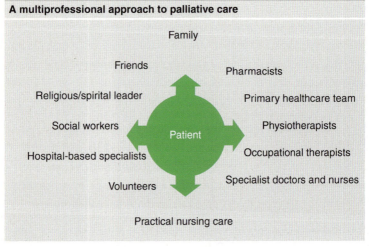

Figure 1.2 A multiprofessional approach to palliative care. (Adapted from O'Neill and Rodway [3])

- attitude to care: a caring attitude, commitment, consideration of individuality, cultural considerations, consent, choice of place of care,
- communication: among healthcare professionals and with patients and families,
- the care: appropriate to the stage of disease, comprehensive and multiprofessional, consistent high standard, coordinated, continuity, crisis prevention, caregiver support and continued reassessment [4], and

- advance care plan: ongoing assessment, multiprofessional meetings, Gold Standards Framework (GSF), Preferred Priorities for Care (PPC), Liverpool Care Pathway (LCP).

Models of Care

In defining and delivering models of care it is important to differentiate the following:

- palliative care principles: these apply to all care, whatever the disease suffered by a patient (Figure 1.3),
- palliative techniques or therapies: include medical and surgical therapies (e.g., stenting, paracentesis, internal fixation of fractures, and radiotherapy) that are employed to palliate symptoms and ease suffering, and
- specialist palliative care (see below) [5].

Categories of Palliative Care Provision

Palliative care is usually provided by two distinct categories of health- and social care professionals, namely those providing the day-to-day care to patients and carers in their homes and in hospitals, and those who specialize in palliative care.

Generalist Palliative Care

Generalist palliative care includes practitioners within primary, secondary, tertiary, and social care and the voluntary sector, many of whom will be specialists in their own sphere of expertise. They will usually assess

---

Palliative care principles

- Affirms life
- Regards dying as a normal process
- Neither hastens nor postpones death
- Provides relief from pain and other distressing symptoms
- Integrates the psychological and spiritual aspects of care
- Offers a support system to help patients live as actively as possible until death
- Offers a support system to help the family cope during the patient's illness and in their own bereavement

Figure 1.3 Palliative care principles. (Data from the World Health Organization [1])

and manage the care needs of each patient and their families across the domains of physical, psychological, social, spiritual, and information needs, and meet those needs within the limits of their knowledge, skills, and competence in palliative care. Generalists should also know when and how to seek advice from or refer to specialist palliative care services.

Specialist Palliative Care

Specialist palliative care includes practitioners who work exclusively within this domain. Specialist palliative care services are usually multi-professional teams comprising, for example, palliative medicine consultants and palliative care nurse specialists, together with a range of expertise provided by physiotherapists, occupational therapists, dieticians, pharmacists, social workers, and those able to give spiritual and psychological support. The service should ideally reflect local practice and needs. In the UK, palliative care is delivered in a number of health-care settings (Figure 1.4) [6]:

- Hospice and palliative care inpatient units: people may sometimes be admitted for inpatient care at an early stage of their illness for a short period of intensive care followed by ongoing support. This could be for rehabilitation following treatment, or for control of symptoms. People may also be admitted to a hospice during the very final stages of their illness. Generally, people stay in an inpatient unit only for a short period of time (perhaps 10–14 days), and will then return to their home or other care setting.

Palliative care services in the UK (2011)	
Service	Number of units
Inpatient units	217
Beds	3194
Day care centers	279
Home care teams	308
Hospital support teams	345
Hospice at home	105

Figure 1.4 Palliative care services in the UK (2011). (Data from Help the Hospices [6])

- Community teams: many people wish to be cared for in their own home. This can be made possible by community palliative care teams that offer specialist care, including advice on pain and symptom control, hands-on nursing, practical advice, and emotional support. The teams can be accessed through district nurses or a person's general practitioner (GP) or family practitioner. Marie Curie nurses provide hands-on, round-the-clock nursing care for people with cancer in their own homes. They are available throughout the UK and their support can be requested by a district nurse. Hospices and palliative care services will provide support for carers in the community too; this may be through a support and information group or by providing one-to-one advice.

- Hospital teams: these teams work alongside surgeons, physicians, nurses, and other health- and social care professionals. Their role is to support the hospital staff by providing education, training, and specialist advice on pain and symptom control. The team will also provide emotional support directly to individuals and their carers, as well as advising staff on planning a patient's discharge home or transfer to another care setting such as a hospice, community hospital, or care home. The team providing this service is sometimes known as a hospital palliative care team, Macmillan support team, or symptom control team. In some hospitals there is a whole team, including doctors, nurses, social workers, and chaplains, whereas in others a single nurse provides the service.

- Day centers: these can give people an opportunity to spend time in a hospice without being an inpatient, allowing them to access the care, and support their needs (including medical, nursing, rehabilitation, creative therapies, complementary therapies) while continuing to live at home.

- Hospice at home: this is usually provided by a multiprofessional team, and they allow people to receive hospice care in their own homes. This may be end-of-life or respite care, or sometimes it may be during a time of crisis. Some teams can offer 24-h nursing care.

Traditionally, hospice and palliative care services were reserved for those with incurable cancer. Increasingly, however, care is provided for other patients with non-cancer illnesses. Moreover, although one-third of the population develop cancer and one-quarter die from it, 75% of the population die from other causes. There are many progressive life-threatening illnesses that reach an end-stage and could benefit from palliative care including heart failure, chronic obstructive pulmonary disease (COPD), and neurological conditions such as multiple sclerosis, motor neuron disease, various dementias, and acquired immune deficiency syndrome (AIDS).

One of the greatest challenges is knowing when the time for palliation has come. The transition from active to palliative therapy is not clear cut and is particularly pertinent in non-cancer diseases because the uncertain disease trajectory can make the decision when to cease active therapy and initiate purely palliative measures difficult (Figure 1.5). Even for patients with cancer, prognostication is inherently difficult and inaccurate despite tools such as the Palliative Performance Scale and the Palliative Prognostic Index [8]. The trend is usually to overestimate prognosis and consequently underestimate planning. The uncertainties impact on both patients and carers, and the question "How long have I got?" may make the clinician feel unprepared to answer effectively (Figure 1.6) [9].

Oncologists often use the Eastern Co-operative Oncology Group (ECOG) score as a measure of patients' functional status (Figure 1.7) [10]. A patient with an ECOG score of more than two, for example, is often deemed to be unsuitable for most chemotherapy treatments.

Supportive Care

Supportive care, a term often used alongside palliative care, helps the patient and family cope with the condition and its treatment, from prediagnosis, through the process of diagnosis and treatment, to cure, continuing illness, or death and into bereavement (Figure 1.8) [11]. Supportive care helps the patient to maximize the benefits of treatment and to live as well as possible with the effects of the disease. It is given equal priority alongside diagnosis and treatment.

The three main trajectories of decline at the end of life

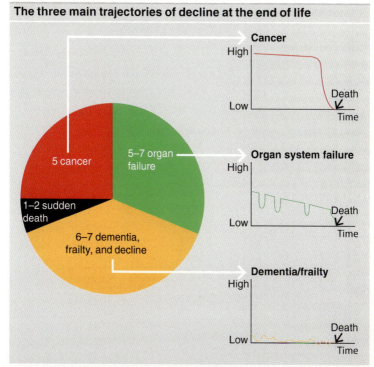

Figure 1.5 The three main trajectories of decline at the end of life. The number of cases of each condition a general practitioner is likely to see per year, with illness trajectories for patients with cancer, organ failure, and old age, frailty, dementia, and decline. (Reproduced with permission from Thomas [7]. © 2006, reproduced with permission from John Wiley and Sons)

Communicating prognosis

- Explain the uncertainty
- Give a realistic timeline
- Provide realistic hope, helping the patient achieve what is important to him or her
- Recommend that family relationships and affairs be attended to
- Be prepared to answer questions about the process of dying
- Provide on-going support and counseling
- Reassure about the continuity of care

Figure 1.6 Communicating prognosis. (Data from Clayton et al. [9])

Supportive care is an 'umbrella' term for generalist and specialist services that may be required to support people with cancer and their carers. It is, therefore, not a distinct specialty, but rather the responsibility of

Eastern Co-operative Oncology Group score

0. Fully active, able to carry on all activities without restriction

1. Restricted in physically strenuous activity but ambulatory and able to carry out work of a light and sedentary nature

2. Ambulatory and capable of all self-care; confined to bed or chair 50% of waking hours

3. Capable of only limited self-care; confined to bed or chair 50% or more of waking hours

4. Completely disabled; cannot carry on any self-care; totally confined to bed or chair

Figure 1.7 Eastern Co-operative Oncology Group score. (Data from Oken et al. [10])

Supportive care

• Self-help and support

• User involvement

• Information giving

• Psychological support

• Symptom control

• Rehabilitation

• Complementary therapies

• Spiritual support

• Palliative care

• End-of-life and bereavement care

Figure 1.8 Supportive care. (Data from the National Institute of Clinical Excellence [11])

all health- and social care professionals delivering care. It requires a spectrum of skills, extending from foundation skills to highly specific expertise and experience. Open and sensitive communication is an important part of supportive care, as is good coordination between and within organizations and teams to ensure the smooth progression of patients from one service to another [11].

Barriers to Palliative Care

Some patients with advanced disease do not receive palliative care. This may be particularly important if complex symptom control or psychosocial issues are present. The reasons for barriers to appropriate palliative care may relate to the physician, the patient, or social factors (Figure 1.9) [5].

In some cases, the patient may have been referred too late in the course of their disease to benefit from treatment, thus adversely affecting

Barriers to palliative care

Physician	Late referral: • Poor prognostication • Lacks the communication skills to address end-of-life issues Reluctant to refer: • Doesn't understand or believe in palliative care • Loss of control, loss of income • Lack of institutional standards for end-of-life care
Patient	Believes that the prognosis is better than what they have been told Unrealistic expectation of disease response Patient–family disagreement about treatment options Lack of advance care plan
Social factors	Ethnic minorities, language barriers Rural communities Poor or underprivileged
Access factors	High cost of care, treatments, and medications in developing countries No government subsidies for healthcare in developing countries No physician reimbursement for palliative care in developing countries Laws and regulations restricting or prohibiting the use of opioids

Figure 1.9 Barriers to palliative care. (Data from Doyle and Woodruff [5])

their end-of-life care. If complex symptom control or psychosocial issues are present or predictable, then advice from or involvement with the specialist palliative care services should be considered.

References

1. World Health Organization. WHO definition of palliative care. www.who.int/cancer/palliative/definition/en. Last accessed 27 Nov 2011.
2. Mount B, Hanks G, McGoldrick L. The principles of palliative care. In: Fallon M, Hanks G, editors. ABC of palliative care. 2nd ed. Oxford: Blackwell Publishing; 2006. p. 1–3.
3. O'Neill B, Rodway A. ABC of palliative care: care in the community. BMJ. 1998;316:373–7.
4. International Association for Hospice and Palliative Care. Manual of palliative care. Available at: www.hospicecare.com/manual/principles-main.html#PRINCIPLES. Last accessed 27 Nov 2011.
5. Doyle D, Woodruff R. The IAHPC manual of palliative care. 2nd ed. Houston: IAHPC Press; 2008. Available at: www.hospicecare.com/manual/IAHPCmanual.htm. Last accessed 27 Nov 2011.
6. Help The Hospices. About hospice care: facts and figures. 2011. www.helpthehospices.org.uk/our-services/information-service. Last accessed 27 Nov 2011.
7. Thomas K. Community palliative care. In: Fallon M, Hanks G, editors. ABC of palliative care. 2nd ed. London: BMJ Books, Blackwell Publishing; 2006. p. 68–73.
8. Glare PA, Sinclair CT. Palliative medicine review: prognostication. J Palliat Med. 2008;11:84–103.

9. Clayton JM, Hancock KM, Butow PN, et al. Clinical practice guidelines for communicating prognosis and end-of-life issues with adults in the advanced stages of a life-limiting illness, and their caregivers. Med J Aust. 2007;186:S77–108.

10. Oken MM, Creech RH, Tormey DC, et al. Toxicity and response criteria of the Eastern Cooperative Oncology Group. Am J Clin Oncol. 1982;5:649–55.

11. National Institute for Clinical Excellence. Improving supportive and palliative care for adults with cancer. London: NICE; 2004.

Chapter 2

Communication Skills

Effective symptom control is impossible without effective communication. Moreover, the success of many clinician–patient relationships depends on our ability to communicate effectively. Effective communication is about conveying information to others clearly and unambiguously. It is also about receiving the information that others are sending. In fact, communication is successful only when both the sender and the receiver understand the same information as a result of the communication (Figure 2.1).

Clinicians need good communication skills to diagnose and treat disease, to establish and maintain a therapeutic relationship, and to offer information and educate. Good communication ensures good working relationships, increases patent satisfaction, increases patient understanding of illness and management, and improves patient adherence to treatment. Good communication can also increase job satisfaction for staff and has similar effects on reducing stress. In a palliative care setting, important and potentially difficult discussions are frequently necessary with patients who have active, progressive, far-advanced disease (Figure 2.2) [1].

Requirements for Effective Communication

Effective communication requires that information is:

- clear,
- concise,
- correct,
- complete,

G. Zeppetella, *Palliative Care in Clinical Practice*,
DOI 10.1007/978-1-4471-2843-4_2,
© Springer-Verlag London 2012

Tips for good communication

- Consider the setting: right place, adequate time, no distractions/interruptions, privacy
- Introduce and greet appropriately
- Show mutual respect
- Use active listening
- Demonstrate empathy
- Acknowledge feelings
- Give each other space
- Maintain appropriate eye contact
- Use language that the patient understands and avoid medical or technical jargon
- Repetition can help people to understand and remember information given to them
- Don't give too much information at one time – only what is needed
- Open, focused questions can encourage patients to talk
- Silence can enable patients to gather their thoughts
- Training can improve your skills in communication

Figure 2.1 Tips for good communication

Examples of potentially difficult discussions

- Breaking bad news
- Further treatment directed at the underlying disease
- Communicating prognoses
- Admission to a hospice
- Artificial nutrition
- Artificial hydration
- Medications such as antibiotics
- Do-not-resuscitate orders

Figure 2.2 Examples of potentially difficult discussions. (Doyle and Woodruff [1])

- courteous, and
- constructive.

Both verbal and non-verbal communication should be congruent. It is sometimes quoted that words are only 7% of the total communication package, whereas tone carries 38% and body language 55% of the overall picture [2]. Congruence is when the words, tone of voice, and body language all convey the same message. Positive body language displays an interest in what the person is saying. For inconsistent messages, or incongruent communications, body language and tonality are probably a more accurate indicator of emotions and meaning than the words themselves.

Throughout the process of communication it is essential to acknowledge that, as healthcare professionals, we have our own agendas, beliefs, and values that can affect the way in which we respond and act with others. Where possible it should be conveyed to the patient and family that they are important and that the aim is to help them. There are many ways to do this [3], and the process should be comfortable and natural. Key characteristics of the process include:

- warmth,
- genuineness,
- empathy,
- acceptance,
- respect,
- dignity,
- trust,
- caring, and
- beliefs and values.

In responding to patients, it is advisable to avoid the following:

- exclamations of surprise, intolerance, or disgust,
- expressions of over-concern,
- moralistic judgments, criticisms, or impatience,
- being defensive and getting caught up in arguments,
- making false promises, giving flattery or undue praise,
- personal references to your own difficulties,
- changing the subject or interrupting unnecessarily, and
- speaking too soon, too often, or for too long.

Verbal Communication

Verbal communication refers to the use of the spoken word to acknowledge, amplify, confirm, contrast, or contradict other verbal and non-verbal messages. Key components of verbal communication include sound, words, speaking, and language (Figure 2.3).

Verbal communication skills

- Let the patient do the talking
- Keep questions brief and simple
- Use language that is understandable to the patient, avoiding acronyms and clinical jargon
- Ask one question at a time, giving the patient time to answer
- Clarify patient responses to questions and let them know that you are listening and that you understand
- Avoid leading questions
- Avoid how or why questions because they tend to be intimidating
- Avoid the use of cliché statements such as, "Don't worry; it'll be all right" or "Your doctor knows best"
- Avoid questions that require only a simple "yes" or "no" response because the aim is to encourage the patient to talk
- Avoid interrupting the patient

Figure 2.3 Verbal communication skills

Active listening

- Maintain eye contact by looking at the speaker
- Stop talking and avoid interrupting
- Sit/stand still, maintaining a body state that reflects attentiveness
- Nod your head to show that you understand
- Lean slightly toward the speaker to show that you are interested
- Check for understanding by repeating information and asking questions for clarification

Figure 2.4 Active listening

Listening

One of the skills required for communication is to listen. Listening means not only hearing what is being said, but also attempting to understand what lies behind the spoken words. Effective listening therefore requires a continuous, determined effort to pay attention to the speaker (Figure 2.4).

Open Questions

Open questions can be answered in any manner and do not direct the respondent or require him or her to make choices from a specific range of answers. They are an essential way of finding out what the patient is experiencing and so help to tailor a support system for the patient. In contrast to open questions, directive (restricts to a predetermined answer), closed (requires the patient to respond yes or no), leading (puts words into patient's mouth), or multiple (questions in quick succession without allowing response from patient) questions are less helpful. For example:

- "How are you feeling?" versus "I suppose you're feeling tired after your treatment."
- "Tell me about your relationship with your partner" versus "Do you have a good relationship with your partner?"
- "What concerns you most about your illness?" versus "Are you concerned that your illness is getting worse?"
- "What has been most difficult about this illness for you?" versus "You must be finding the illness difficult?"

Silence

Silence is a technique for facilitating dialogue between a patient and clinician. If the patient is speaking, do not talk over him or her. Waiting for the patient to stop speaking before replying is a simple, but often ignored, rule most likely to give patients the impression that they are not being listened to. Silences also have other meanings. Often a patient falls silent when he or she has feelings too intense to express in words. A silence, therefore, means that the patient is thinking or feeling something important, not that he or she has stopped thinking. If you need to break the silence, a helpful way to do so is to say: "What were you thinking about just then?" or "What is making you pause?" Silence also gives the clinician time to think and assimilate what has been said.

Non-verbal Communication

Non-verbal communication is the process of communicating through gesture, body language or posture, facial expression, and eye contact (Figure 2.5) [4]. Speech may also contain non-verbal elements including voice quality, emotion, and speaking style, as well as rhythm, intonation, and stress. Other techniques can involve:

- acknowledgment/facilitation,
- encouragement,
- picking up cues,

Using posture to communicate	
S	Sit square to the patient
O	Open to the patient
L	Lean in toward the patient
E	Eye contact with the patient
R	Relax

Figure 2.5 **Using posture to communicate**. (Data from Egan [4])

Reasons for poor communication	
Patients	Language barriers
	Fear of getting upset/emotional
	Tiredness/illness
	Feeling like a burden/taking up too much time
	Consider staff too busy or not interested
Staff	Language barriers
	Not knowing what to say
	Fear of dealing with strong emotions
	Not knowing enough

Figure 2.6 **Reasons for poor communication**

- reflection,
- clarification, and
- empathy.

Barriers to Effective Communication

Poor communication and information giving are some of the most common causes for complaints. This may be as a result of factors related to either the patient or the healthcare professional (Figure 2.6).

Recognizing the barriers is the first step to effective communication (Figure 2.7). Remember too that the interpersonal gap is the difference between the backgrounds, education, religious beliefs, and history of each party and how clearly each understands the other.

Effective communication, both verbally and non-verbally, is an essential element of any generalist or specialist clinician's management strategy, "seek first to understand, then to be understood" [5]. Gain an understanding of the patients' fears, expectations, hopes, and concerns,

Barriers to good communication
- Lack of time
- Lack of privacy
- Uncertainty
- Embarrassment
- Collusion
- Maintaining hope
- Anger
- Denial

Figure 2.7 Barriers to good communication

where they are 'coming from.' It is only through a common understanding of the problem that a common solution can be explored with both the patient and the family.

Further Reading

Rungapadiachy DM. Interpersonal communication and psychology for health care professionals: theory and practice. London: Butterworth Heinemann; 1999.

References

1. Doyle D, Woodruff R. The IAHPC manual of palliative care. 2nd ed. Houston: IAHPC Press; 2008. Available at: www.hospicecare.com/manual/IAHPCmanual.htm. Last accessed 27 Nov 2011.
2. Mehrabian A. Silent messages: implicit communication of emotions and attitudes. Belmont: Wadsworth; 1981.
3. Oken MM, Creech RH, Tormey DC, et al. Toxicity and response criteria of the Eastern Cooperative Oncology Group. Am J Clin Oncol. 1982;5:649–55.
4. Egan G. The skilled helper: a problem-management and opportunity-development approach to helping. 9th ed. Pacific Grove: Thomson Brooks/Cole; 2007.
5. Covey SR. The seven habits of highly effective people. New York: Fireside Books, Simon & Schuster; 1990.

Chapter 3

Breaking Bad News

Bad news is defined as any news that seriously and negatively alters the patient's view of his or her future. In trying to convey the news as sensitively as possible, it is essential to help the patient and the family understand the condition, support the patient and family, and minimize the risk of overwhelming distress or prolonged denial:

> The task of breaking bad news is a testing ground for the entire range of our professional skills and abilities. If we do it badly, the patients or family members may never forgive us; if we do it well, they will never forget us [1].

Bad news situations can include disease recurrence, spread of disease, failure of treatment to affect disease progression, the presence of irreversible side effects, or raising the issue of palliative care and resuscitation. The principles of breaking bad news are applicable to all situations, including information given to relatives, although it should be remembered that all information given to the relatives of competent adults should be done only with the patient's permission.

Patients often have vivid memories of receiving bad news, and negative experiences can have lasting effects on anxiety and depression. If done well, breaking bad news can facilitate adaptation to illness and deepen the relationship between the patient and healthcare professional. Yet clinicians often dislike giving bad news because of the fear of causing more harm or feeling blamed for the "bad news." There may be a sense of

G. Zeppetella, *Palliative Care in Clinical Practice*,
DOI 10.1007/978-1-4471-2843-4_3,
© Springer-Verlag London 2012

failing the patients and of feeling helpless and embarrassed. A number of factors can affect a doctor's ability to impart bad news sensitively, including burnout and fatigue, personal difficulties, behavioral beliefs, subjective attitudes, and prior clinical experience.

Steps to Breaking Bad News

The key to breaking bad news well is to ensure the transition from patients' perceptions that they are well to a realization that they have a life-threatening or life-changing disease. If the news is given too abruptly, the patient may have difficulty adapting psychologically. Moreover, you don't often need to tell people, they usually tell you if you allow them. In reality, patients appreciate concern and empathy, and feelings expressed are more likely to be therapeutic rather than damaging. There are several strategies for breaking bad news that may be helpful (Figures 3.1 and 3.2).

Difficult reactions may follow the imparting of bad news such as silence, anger, and denial. It is good practice for a staff member to stay with the patient after the bad news has been given, to provide support and allow the patient an opportunity to express his or her thoughts. Further follow-up may be necessary to ensure that the patient has absorbed and retained the information. It is important throughout to document what the patient has been told and what follow-up arrangements have been made.

Ten steps to breaking bad news
1. Preparation
2. What is known?
3. Is more information wanted?
4. Allow denial
5. The warning shot
6. Explain
7. Listen to concern
8. Ventilation of feelings
9. Summarize and make a plan
10. Offer availability

Figure 3.1 Ten steps to breaking bad news. (Data from Kaye [2])

BREAKING BAD NEWS · 21

Breaking bad news – a guide for clinical staff

Guidance	Notes
Prepare yourself	Familiarize yourself with the patient's background, medical history, test results, and future management/treatment choices
	Mentally rehearse the interview, including likely questions and potential responses
	Arrange for a colleague such as the patient's named nurse or specialist nurse to accompany you. Relatives can be in attendance; however, you must be guided by the wishes of the patient
Prepare your setting	Arrange some privacy
	Do not stand over the patient; sit down because this relaxes the patient and shows that you are not going to be rushed. If you have recently examined the patient, allow him or her to dress before the interview
	Switch your pager off or get a colleague to answer calls on your behalf
Prepare your patient	Assess patients' understanding of their condition. "Can you help me by telling me what you understand about your illness?"
	Although many patients want to have details about their disease and diagnosis, some patients do not want this detail and their wishes should be respected and appropriately managed. Never impose information
Provide information	Start at the level of comprehension and vocabulary of the patient
	Use non-technical words such as "spread" instead of "metastases"
	Avoid excessive bluntness, because it is likely to leave the patienti isolated and later angry
	Set the tone. "I am afraid I have some bad news"
	Give the information in small chunks and stop periodically to check the patient's understanding. "Is this making sense?" or "Would you like me to explain more?" When the prognosis is poor, avoid using terms such as "There is nothing more we can do for you," because goals in care will change to pain control and symptom relief
Provide support	Acknowledge and identify with the emotion experienced by the patient. When patients are silent, use open questions, asking them how they are feeling or thinking. This will help them articulate what their emotions are. "How are you feeling now?"
	Do not say? "i know how you feel." Even if you have had personal experience of the disease or condition, you cannot know how an individual feels. Empathy can be shown by using terms such as, "I think I understand how you must be feeling"
	Allow patients time to express their emotions and let them know that you understand and acknowledge their emotions
	Unless a patient's emotions are adequately addressed, it is difficult for the doctor and patient to move on to discuss other important issues but remember that the patient's crisis is not your crisis – listen

Figure 3.2 Breaking bad news – a guide for clinical staff (continues overleaf).

Breaking bad news – a guide for clinical staff	
Guidance	Notes
Provide a plan	Provide a clear plan for the future, with treatment options or management plan discussed
	Offer to meet and talk to the family if not present
After the interview	Make a clear record of the interview, the terms used, the options discussed, and the future plan. Ensure that the detail of the interview is shared with the multidisciplinary team, including the general practitioner or family practitioner

Figure 3.2 Breaking bad news – a guide for clinical staff (continued). (Reproduced with permission from the National Council for Hospice and Specialist Palliative Care Services [3])

Dealing with False Hope

Patients should always be informed of the situation in a truthful way, because honesty will strengthen the relationship with the patient, and improve cooperation and their ability to cope as the disease progresses. Important information should, however, be delivered in a tactful manner, supporting the patient (relying on acknowledgment and exploration of the patient's feelings), and delivered at the patient's pace and in a way that will enable the clinician to recruit and reinforce instead of diminishing the patient's coping strategies to face the situation.

A frequently heard response from carers and clinicians alike is "You can't take away hope." It should be considered whether the rationale behind this has more to do with protecting the clinician from discomfort than protecting the patient. Moreover, many patients with advanced illness and their carers prefer disclosure, and patients who know their prognosis have been shown to have a lower rate of emotional distress and higher health-related quality of life [4]. Insensitive and ineffective truth telling may be just as damaging and counterproductive as insensitive lying.

The issue with bad news is that it is bad! It can have the potential to shatter hopes and dreams. Breaking bad news is a complex task that requires expert verbal and non-verbal skills. Through careful planning preparation, support, and follow-up we may be able to lessen the impact and help patients and their families cope with the consequences of the news. At the very least we should not make the situation worse through our own fears, apprehensions, misconceptions, and lack of training.

References

1. Buckman R, Kason Y. How to break bad news: a guide for health care professionals. Baltimore: Johns Hopkins University Press; 1992.
2. Kaye P. Breaking bad news. Northampton: EPL Publications; 1996.
3. National Council for Hospice and Specialist Palliative Care Services. Regional Guidelines on Breaking Bad News. Published by Department of Health, Social Services & Public Safety, Belfast Last accessed 16 April 2012 http://www.dhsspsni.gov.uk/breaking_bad_news.pdf
4. Yun YH, Kwon YC, Lee MK, et al. Experiences and attitudes of patients with terminal cancer and their family caregivers towards the discussion of terminal illness. J Clin Oncol. 2010;28:1950–7.

Chapter 4

Symptom Control

Symptoms are the patient's perceptions of abnormal physiological changes due to the disease or its treatment. As symptoms are dynamic and can change over time, their management is central to the practice of palliative care. It is important to make a diagnosis of the underlying mechanisms or causes of the symptom, individualize the treatment, and, where possible, keep the management simple (Figure 4.1).

Prevalent Symptoms in Palliative Care Patients

In a retrospective case note review of 400 consecutive referrals to palliative care services, the five most prevalent symptoms were pain, anorexia, constipation, weakness, and dyspnea with patients presenting with, on average, up to 27 different symptoms (Figure 4.2) [1]. The complex

Management principles	
Evaluation	Always assess for the cause of symptoms
Explanation	Give a good clear explanation of the mechanism underlying the symptom, the treatment options, and the involvement of the family
Individualized treatment	The patient should determine the treatment priorities, and realistic goals should be set in partnership with patients
Supervision	Regular monitoring of symptom control is needed to ensure that dosage is optimum,adverse effects are avoided or minimized, and treatment goals are being met

Figure 4.1 Management principles

G. Zeppetella, *Palliative Care in Clinical Practice*,
DOI 10.1007/978-1-4471-2843-4_4,
© Springer-Verlag London 2012

Prevalence of symptoms in patients referred to palliative care services

Percentage referrals with symptom

Symptom	All (n=400)	Hospice (n=100)	Community (n=100)	Hospital (n=100)	Outpatient (n=100)
Pain	64	62	56	63	75
Anorexia*	34	58	56	6	17
Constipation*	32	52	35	22	17
Weakness	32	41	73	5	10
Dyspnea*	31	50	41	18	13
Nausea	29	37	34	25	18
Neuropsychiatric	27	39	28	28	11
Tiredness	23	24	42	7	18
Weight loss	18	12	46	3	10
Low mood	16	10	27	10	15
Vomiting	16	24	5	22	13
Dry mouth	16	31	26	2	5
Cough	15	30	18	8	5
Dermatological	14	35	16	0	7
Urinary	14	19	29	2	5
Anxiety	13	15	17	7	13
Edema	12	18	14	3	13
Sleep problem	12	22	24	0	2
Loose stool	10	10	17	5	6
Dyspepsia	8	14	8	0	8
Numbness/tingling	8	9	18	1	5
Dysphagia	7	11	8	3	5
Hemorrhage	6	4	7	9	5
Early satiety	4	1	12	3	0
Sweating	3	5	2	0	4
Hiccoughs	2	0	6	1	0
Taste change	2	1	6	0	0

Figure 4.2 Prevalence of symptoms in patients referred to palliative care services.
*Statistical significance of symptom prevalence between the groups: $P < 0.001$. (Data from Potter et al. [1]. Reproduced with permission from SAGE)

nature of the symptoms, their subjectivity, and the enormous variability in individual perceptions, evaluations, and responses necessitates that the management of these problems typically requires a multifaceted and individualized response.

Symptom Assessment and Management

Each patient has a right to symptom assessment and symptom management including:

- individualized approach,
- comprehensive assessment,
- effective communication,
- education and reassurance,
- encouragement of participation, and
- comprehensive reassessment.

Symptom assessment should be provided systematically and regularly in clinical practice and many appropriate assessment tools are available [2]. The cancer itself is not always the direct cause of the symptom. A useful framework when assessing symptoms is, therefore, to consider causal factors as related to:

- disease,
- treatment,
- debility, and
- concurrent disorder.

Basic symptom control should be initiated by those providing general palliative care. For many patients in the late stages of their illness, the palliative care needs are straightforward and can be met by the primary care and/or specialist team. However, if complex symptom control or psychosocial issues are present or predictable, then advice from or involvement with the specialist palliative care services should be considered.

Symptom control guidelines, either local or national, should be followed with clear indications for referral to specialist palliative care services if symptoms are not rapidly controlled. This chapter provides a brief management strategy for common symptoms in palliative care patients.

Anemia
Definition

Anemia is defined as a hemoglobin (Hb) of <11.5 g/L in females and <13.5 g/L in males. In a palliative care population a lower Hb is considered clinically significant.

Prevalence

Anemia has been described in up to 73% of hospice inpatients [3]. The cause may be multifactorial, including anemia of chronic disease, acute or chronic hemorrhage, bone marrow suppression or invasion, malnutrition, or hemolysis [3]. Anemia is more common in patients with leukemia, lymphoma, lung, or gynecological and gastrointestinal (GI) cancers. The following are causes of anemia in palliative care patients [4]:

- marrow failure/suppression,
- anemia of chronic disease,
- acute and chronic hemorrhage,
- hemolysis,
- malnutrition, and
- underlying chronic or congenital anemia.

Assessment

The symptoms of anemia include:

- tiredness,
- weakness,
- breathlessness on exertion,
- postural hypotension, and
- edema.

Although patients may have symptoms that might be attributable to anemia, the low Hb may also be due to their underlying disease [4]. Consequently, the management of these patients requires that the benefits and burdens of investigation and treatment be considered.

The symptoms of anemia also depend on how quickly the Hb drops. Patients may tolerate lower levels if they have had time to develop chronic compensatory mechanisms, such as an increase in heart and respiratory rates and reduced systemic vascular resistance. These adaptations decrease symptoms by improving oxygenation.

Diagnosis of anemia requires routine hematological investigations, including Hb and mean corpuscular volume measurements. Anemia is frequently mild and normocytic, indicating a most likely diagnosis of anemia of chronic disease, which should be distinguished from iron deficiency anemia (Figure 4.3) [6].

Discriminating between anemias

	Anemia of chronic disease	Iron deficiency anemia
Hemoglobin	7–11 g/dL	↓
MCV	N or↓	Usually↓ (<76 fL)
Ferritin	N or ↑	↑
Serum iron	N or↓	↓
Total iron-binding capacity	N or↓	↑
Transferrin receptor levels	N	↑
Bone marrow	Iron stores↑↑	No iron stores

Figure 4.3 Discriminating between anemias. ↓ decreased, ↑ increased, *MCV* mean corpuscular volume, *N* normal. (Data from Hirst [5]. Reproduced with permission from MIMS)

Iron content of different iron salts

Preparation	Dose (mg)	Iron content (mg)
Ferrous fumarate	200	65
Ferrous gluconate	300	35
Ferrous sulfate	300	60
Ferrous sulfate, dried	200	65

Figure 4.4 Iron content of different iron salts. (Reproduced with permission from the British National Formulary [7]. Reproduced with permission from the Joint Formulary Committee)

General Management

Anemia may be an indicator of a poor prognosis in itself. If the anemia is mild, no treatment may be necessary or helpful, whatever the underlying cause.

Pharmacological Management

Iron

Iron therapy is particularly used in patients with a longer prognosis. The patient should be warned that bowel motions become black, and that adverse effects include constipation or diarrhea. Several iron preparations are available (Figure 4.4) [7].

Ferrous sulfate 200 mg tds or ferrous gluconate 300 mg four to six tablets daily in divided doses before food should be prescribed. It would be reasonable to expect a rise in Hb of 1–2 g/L every 3 weeks with oral iron. Parenteral iron does not result in a faster rise, except in patients on hemodialysis, but it does replenish body stores more rapidly.

Vitamin B12

Vitamin B12 preparations may be used when iron deficiency exists. It is usually given with a folate supplement because a deficiency in both is possible. The dose is initially 1 mg three times a week for 2 weeks, followed by a maintenance dose of 1 mg every month.

Erythropoietin

Erythropoietin is not commonly used in palliative care because, although early studies seemed to show that erythropoietin reduced the need for blood transfusions, raised Hb, and improved quality of life in patients receiving cancer treatment, there are associated risks such as an increased number of thrombotic events [8].

Non-pharmacological Management

Blood Transfusion

Many palliative care facilities in the UK will consider blood transfusions for a patient whose Hb drops below 8 g/dL [9]. Nevertheless, it is important to treat the patient, and not the blood results. For example, an elderly patient with ischemic heart disease may need to be transfused at a higher Hb if angina occurs at rest. Indications for a blood transfusion include the following:

- symptomatic due to anemia,
- anemia of gradual onset,
- Hb <8 g/L, and
- weakness and fatigue can contribute to anemia rather than advancing it and the disease improvement with blood transfusion may be only transient (i.e., 1–2 days).

Patients should be reassessed 1 week after the transfusion for any symptom relief. If pretransfusion symptoms, such as fatigue and dyspnea, are not improved after this time, further transfusions are unlikely to help.

Anorexia

Definition

Anorexia/cachexia syndrome (ACS) is a complex metabolic process found in many end-stage illnesses, characterized by a loss of appetite, weight loss, and tissue wasting.

Prevalence

ACS affects up to 80% of patients with advanced cancer and causes both physical and psychological distress [10]. Primary ACS results from a hypermetabolic state caused directly by the cancer. Secondary ACS results from cancer-related barriers that reduce, for example, dietary intake, such as nausea/vomiting, mucositis, and changes in taste/smell from chemotherapy. ACS is often associated with other symptoms, including early satiety, fatigue, and a change in body image.

Assessment

Assessment of ACS should include the following:
- exclusion of reversible causes (e.g., pain, depression, nausea, vomiting, constipation, and dysphagia),
- exclusion of exacerbating factors (e.g., odors, delayed gastric emptying),
- check for oral problems (e.g., xerostomia, ill-fitting dentures, ulcers, candidiasis),
- find out about the patient and caregiver perspectives on weight, body image, nutrition, dietary intake, and
- assessment of the psychosocial aspects.

General Management

The prevention or early identification and treatment of contributory symptoms are important strategies [11]. The psychological impact on the patient and caregiver should be acknowledged, and ongoing discussion and support are needed. Supplementary drinks can help selected patients after a careful assessment of nutritional status, prognosis, and alternative options.

Pharmacological Management

Medication may be of limited benefit, but worth considering.

Corticosteroids

Although corticosteroids have been shown to significantly improve appetite, caloric intake, energy/wellbeing, and functional status, they do not impact weight [12]. Due to the consequences of long-term use (beyond 4 weeks), they are limited in use, but they may be beneficial in improving the quality of life in patients with a limited prognosis. Common dosing for primary ACS has been the equivalent of dexamethasone 4 mg; however, the ideal dosing or choice of corticosteroid has not been established.

Corticosteroids for anorexia [13]:

- have an established role in short-term improvement of appetite,
- have a rapid effect, which tends to decrease after 3–4 weeks,
- may also reduce nausea, and improve energy/general feeling of wellbeing, and
- have no significant effect on nutritional status.

In addition:

- Starting dose: oral dexamethasone 4 mg or prednisolone 30 mg in the morning. Consider the need for a proton pump inhibitor (PPI).
- Consider and explain adverse effects (e.g., fluid retention, candidiasis, myopathy, insomnia, gastritis).
- Prescribe for 1 week and, if there is no benefit, stop. If helpful, reduce to the lowest effective dose. Review regularly and withdraw if no longer improving symptoms.

Progestogens

Progestogens have been one of the major treatments for primary ACS and have the most evidence for weight gain and improved appetite in cancer patients [12]. Progestogens for anorexia [13]:

- improve appetite and increase weight in patients with cancer,
- take a few weeks to take effect but benefits more prolonged than steroids, and
- more appropriate for patients with a longer prognosis.

In addition:

- Megestrol acetate – starting dose 160 mg orally daily for 1 month, then review.
- Dose range: 160–800 mg; no evidence for optimal dose.
- Side effects: nausea, fluid retention, increased risk of thromboembolism.

- Reduce dose gradually if used for more than 3 weeks (adrenal suppression).

Megestrol acetate increases weight, primarily in fat, rather than lean body mass. Although studies have demonstrated a symptomatic improvement of appetite, caloric intake, and general wellbeing at doses as low as 180 mg, the ideal dosing for weight gain is in the range 480–800 mg daily [14]. Medroxyprogesterone acetate is used in similar circumstances because doses of progestogens may result in an increased risk of thrombosis. Caution should therefore be taken in patients with cancer who have a prior history of thrombosis. Other possible side effects include peripheral edema, hypertension, hyperglycemia, breakthrough uterine bleeding, and suppression of the hypothalamic–pituitary–adrenal axis.

Other

Prokinetics can be used for early satiety, delayed gastric emptying, gastroparesis, or nausea. A trial of metoclopramide 10 mg or domperidone 10–20 mg (fewer long-term side effects) given three times daily half an hour before meals should be considered. Low doses of dronabinol have been shown to simulate appetite, an effect that may be related to the mood-altering effects of this group of drugs [12].

Non-pharmacological Management

The concerns of the patient and caregiver about the importance of giving nourishment, refusing food, and eating as a social activity should be addressed. Explanations should be given on the fact that gradual reduction in oral intake is a natural part of the illness and information needs to be offered and practical advice given about nutrition in advanced illness, as well as diet and management of anorexia.

Patient and Caregiver Advice Points

The patient should be gently encouraged to take what nourishment he or she can manage. Soft, easy-to-swallow foods such as soup, pudding, nutritious drinks, or snacks should be offered in small, attractively presented portions more often through the day. It is advisable to try not to talk about food all the time but keep the patient involved in the social aspects of meals.

Anxiety
Definition
Anxiety is a state of apprehension and fear resulting from the perception of a current or future threat to oneself.

Prevalence
Anxiety is a common symptom for those facing life-threatening ill-nesses. At least 25% of cancer patients experience significant anxiety, of which at least 3% meet the *Diagnostic and Statistical Manual of Mental Disorders* (DSM) criteria for generalized anxiety disorder [15, 16]. Patients are often faced with a number of somatic symptoms, as well as recurrent unpleasant thoughts including fears of pain, death, and dependency on others [17]. The following are anxiety symptoms in can-cer patients:

- restlessness,
- worry, foreboding, apprehension,
- panic symptoms:
  - palpitations, tachycardia,
  - sweating,
  - breathlessness,
  - GI distress and nausea,
  - feelings of impending doom,
- difficulty falling asleep or awakening in the middle of the night, and
- irritability.

Assessment
Anxiety may be present as part of one or several psychiatric disorders, including generalized anxiety disorder, panic disorder, adjustment disor-der, acute- or post-traumatic stress disorder, or phobias. The diagnosis of anxiety in the palliative care setting is usually determined by questions asked in a clinical interview:

- "Do you feel nervous or jittery?"
- "Have you felt fearful, distressed, or tense? Of anything in particular?"
- "Do you avoid certain activities or people because of fear?"
- "Have you felt a lump in your throat or a knot in the pit of your stomach when getting upset?"
- "Are you afraid to close your eyes at night for fear that you will die in your sleep?"
- "Are you often worried about what death or dying will be like?"

In the palliative care setting it may be difficult to distinguish the somatic causes of anxiety from the psychological ones. The following are some possible causes of anxiety in cancer patients [17]:

- poor pain control,
- metabolic:
  - hypoxia,
  - delirium,
  - sepsis,
  - bleeding,
  - pulmonary embolus,
  - hypocalcemia,
  - nutritional failure,
- drug induced:
  - corticosteroids,
  - antiemetics,
  - bronchodilators, and
  - substances abuse or withdrawal (e.g., alcohol, opioids, benzodiazepines).

Several instruments have been used to measure anxiety including the Hospital Anxiety and Depression Scale (HADS), which is a self-report measure that assesses the cognitive items associated with depression and anxiety [18], and the distress thermometer, which is a one-item visual analog scale in the form of a thermometer that may be a more feasible screening tool in the palliative care setting (see Appendix 2) [19].

General Management

A patient's anxiety may be prevented or alleviated by emotional support and information, together with an exploration of their fears about disease progression, psychosocial difficulties, and death. Patients should have opportunities to express their feelings if they are to move on toward accepting their circumstances.

Pharmacological Management

Benzodiazepines are the first-line anxiolytics for the patient who has felt persistently apprehensive and anxious (Figure 4.5) [19]. For patients with compromised hepatic function, the use of shorter-acting

Drugs used to treat anxiety			
Class	Drug	Approximate daily dose (mg)	Routes
Benzodiazepines	Midazolam	10–60 q24h	iv, sc
	Alprazolam	0.25–2.0 tds/qds	po, sl
	Oxazepam	10–15 tds/qds	po
	Lorazepam	0.2–2.0 tds/qds	po, sl, iv
	Chlordiazepoxide	10–50 tds/qds	po
	Diazepam	5–10 bd/qds	po, iv, pr
	Clonazepam	0.5–2.0 bd/qds	po
Non-benzodiazepines	Buspirone	5.0–20 tds	po
Neuroleptics	Haloperidol	0.5–5.0 q2–12h	po, iv, sc
	Levomepromazine	10–20 q4–8h	po, sc, iv
	Chlorpromazine	12.5–50 q4–12h	po, iv
Atypical neuroleptics	Olanzapine	2.5–20 q12–24h	po
	Risperidone	1.3–3.0 q12–24h	po
Antihistamine	Hydroxyzine	25–50 q4–6h	po, sc, iv
Tricyclic antidepressants	Imipramine	12.5–150 daily	po
	Clomipramine	10–150 daily	po

Figure 4.5 **Drugs used to treat anxiety**. *bd* twice daily, *iv* intravenously, *po* orally, *pr* rectally, *qds* four times daily, *sc* subcutaneously, *sl* sublingually, *tds* three times daily. (Data from Breitbart et al. [20])

benzodiazepines, such as lorazepam and oxazepam for anxiety and temazepam for sleep, is preferred. A longer-acting benzodiazepine, such as clonazepam, may provide more consistent relief of anxiety symptoms and may also have mood-stabilizing effects [17]. For insomnia, the benzodiazepine temazepam, as well as the non-benzodiazepine hypnotic zolpidem may be effective. Buspirone, a 5-hydroxytryptamine (5HT1) agonist, is indicated for use in generalized anxiety. It is less sedating than the benzodiazepines, but has a slower onset of action (at least 2 weeks) and can cause nausea in some patients.

For the management of panic disorder the benzodiazepines alprazolam and clonazepam and antidepressant medications (i.e., selective serotonin reuptake inhibitors [SSRIs], tricyclic antidepressants [TCAs], and monoamine oxidase inhibitors [MAOIs]) have demonstrated effectiveness. Alprazolam rapidly blocks panic attacks. The TCA imipramine is effective in the management of panic disorder. Its anticholinergic side effects are, however, not well tolerated by all patients.

Non-pharmacological Management

Psychotherapy aims to increase the individual's sense of his or her own wellbeing through a range of techniques based on experiential relationship building, dialogue, communication, and behavior. Two of the most effective forms of psychotherapy used to treat anxiety disorders are behavioral therapy and cognitive–behavioral therapy [21].

Behavioral Therapy

Behavioral therapy helps unlearn self-defeating patterns and habits and teaches new, healthy skills and ways of reacting to situations that trigger anxiety. Behavioral therapy is action based, and assumes that, if the patient can learn to change his or her behavior, thoughts, feelings, and attitudes will change too. Behavioral strategies may include progressive muscle relaxation techniques, gradual exposure to the anxiety trigger, changing breathing patterns, positive and negative reinforcement, and learning empowering ways of relating to others.

Cognitive Therapy

Cognitive therapy assumes that, by changing self-defeating thought patterns (e.g., all-or-nothing beliefs, negative assumptions, labeling), and transforming them into more successful belief systems, patients can improve their mental and emotional health.

Cognitive–Behavioral Therapy

Cognitive–behavioral therapy is a combination approach that uses both cognitive and behavioral therapy. These two therapies complement each other and, when used together, they stimulate areas of growth that are difficult to achieve using one or the other by itself. Cognitive–behavioral therapy addresses both the thoughts and the behaviors that promote and perpetuate anxiety.

Ascites
Definition

Ascites is defined as the pathological accumulation of fluid in the abdominal cavity.

Prevalence

Approximately 10% of all cases of ascites are caused by cancer and 15–50% of all cancer patients will develop ascites [22]. The usual causes of ascites are malignancies of the GI tract (carcinoma of stomach, colon, and pancreas, primary hepatocellular carcinoma, and metastatic liver cancer), carcinoma of the ovary, Hodgkin's lymphoma and non-Hodgkin's lymphoma, and metastatic carcinoma within the abdominal cavity. The presence of ascites tends to suggest widespread disease and a poor prognosis [23].

Assessment

A small amount of fluid in the abdominal cavity is normal and helps to lubricate the surfaces of the peritoneum. For fluid to be detectable by clinical examination there has to be at least 1,500 mL present, slightly less in a small, thin person, but significantly more in obese individuals, whereas ultrasonography can detect much smaller volumes (≤500 mL).

Shifting dullness is used to detect ascites:

1. Percuss from the level of the umbilicus and repeat moving laterally toward one side.
2. When the sound becomes dull, keep your fingers there to mark the spot and ask the patient to move on to the opposite side.
3. Wait briefly for the fluid to sink and percuss again. If it is now resonant, that is a positive sign.
4. Percuss down until dullness is reached again.
5. Repeat on the other side.

A succussion splash is much more difficult to demonstrate. It needs a third hand in the examination and probably rather more fluid.

General Management

Mild ascites may not require any specific treatment, but should be regularly monitored. Patients should be advised of what to expect and when to seek further advice.

Pharmacological Management

Spironolactone is usually the first-choice treatment, because it increases sodium excretion and potassium reabsorption in the distal tubules; 100 mg/day can gradually be increased to 400 mg/day as necessary. Serum potassium levels need monitoring because hyperkalemia frequently limits spironolactone's use [24].

Loop diuretics may be used as an adjunct to spironolactone, generally only when maximum doses of the latter have been reached. Start cautiously with, for example, furosemide 40 mg/day, although up to 160 mg/day may be used. High doses cause severe electrolyte disturbance, particularly hyponatremia [24].

Non-pharmacological Management

Paracentesis is a simple technique that can be used for diagnostic or therapeutic purposes. As a palliative procedure it can provide good, although temporary, relief of abdominal pain, breathlessness, nausea, vomiting, and dyspepsia. Patients with large or refractory ascites generally benefit most. Paracentesis is contraindicated if the patient is unable to cooperate or has a skin infection at the proposed puncture site, severe bowel distension, or coagulopathy [24].

Peritoneovenous shunts may be appropriate in a minority of patients who have recurrent ascites, although their use has to be balanced by the potential risks of the procedure. Patients will have usually demonstrated transient symptomatic improvement with paracentesis. Commonly used shunts include the LeVeen and Denver shunts, which direct fluid from the abdominal cavity into the vena cava. A unidirectional valve ensures that the ascites can flow only from the peritoneum into the vein.

Other options include systemic or intraperitoneal chemotherapy, intraperitoneal radiotherapy, and intraperitoneal immunotherapy.

Breathlessness
Definition
Breathlessness is defined as difficult, distressing breathing.

Prevalence
Breathlessness is reported in approximately 50% of all cancer patients; in patients with lung cancer the prevalence is 70% and rises in the final weeks of life [25]. It impacts on physical function, other physical symptoms, emotional problems, social function, existential issues, and coping ability.

Assessment
Breathlessness is subjective and may correlate poorly with objective assessment of lung function, including blood gas analysis and airway obstruction [26]. The causes of breathlessness may be related to the cancer or cancer treatment, or be independent of them (Figure 4.6). During the course of the assessment it is important to:

- Clarify the pattern of breathlessness (e.g., continuous, intermittent, resting, exertional, paroxysmal).
- Determine if there are any precipitating/alleviating factors and associated symptoms.
- Elucidate whether treatment of the underlying disease is appropriate.
- Look for any reversible causes of breathlessness.

Causes of breathlessness	
Cancer	Effusions
	Obstruction to main bronchus
	Replacement of lung tissue
	Lymphangitis
	Superior vena cava obstruction
	Pericardial effusions
	Ascites
Cancer therapies	Pneumonectomy
	Radiation fibrosis
	Chemotherapy
Debility	Anemia
	Atelectasis
	Pulmonary embolus
	Pneumonia
	Empyema
Other causes	Chronic obstructive pulmonary disease
	Asthma
	Heart failure
	Acidosis
	Painful chest lesions
	Respiratory muscle dysfunction

Figure 4.6 Causes of breathlessness

- Check oxygen saturation.
- Ask the patient to rate symptom severity and level of associated distress/anxiety.
- Explore fears, impact on functional abilities, and quality of life.
- Avoid unnecessary investigation: consider the stage of disease, previous treatment, and wishes of the patient and family.

General Management

The general management of breathlessness involves the following:

- Treat any reversible causes, if appropriate.
- Encourage modification of lifestyle in reducing non-essential activities, while trying to maintain mobility and independence as far as possible.
- Encourage exertion to the point of breathlessness to build tolerance and maintain fitness; this varies considerably between individuals; pulmonary rehabilitation is increasingly considered in a palliative setting.

- Teach the use of breathing exercises and relaxation methods.
- Modify the diet, with small frequent drinks and meals being best tolerated.
- Ensure that the patient is in the most comfortable position, usually sitting upright with support.
- Keep the room cool and use a fan or open window.
- Pay attention to oral hygiene. Mouth breathing dries the mouth and oxygen will be very dry unless it has been humidified.

Pharmacological Management

Opioids

Oral and parenteral opioids can reduce breathlessness, particularly at rest and in the terminal phase, and the risk of significant respiratory depression is much less than anticipated [27]. Oral morphine is widely used to manage breathlessness and the patient should be started on a low dose as a therapeutic trial, and titrated according to response and adverse effects. Patients not already receiving morphine should start at doses of 5 mg q4h prn (lower doses should be used in frail or elderly patients, and in patients with impaired renal function). For patients already on morphine, whether for pain or dyspnea, the overall dose may need to be increased by 30–50%. When the oral route is no longer available, administration by continuous subcutaneous infusion (CSCI) has been shown to be effective.

Anxiolytics

Anxiolytics are commonly used to treat breathlessness in palliative care, although the literature suggests that their use should be second line or third line on an individual therapeutic trial basis [28]. Diazepam, lorazepam, and midazolam are most frequently used. It is usual to start with a low dose and increase gradually as required and tolerated. Selection depends on the stage of terminal disease, the severity of the anxiety, and the desired onset of action. Lorazepam can be administered 0.5 mg sl, as required, for episodic anxiety, panic attacks, or alternatively diazepam 5 mg at night if the patient is experiencing more continuous anxiety. TCAs and SSRIs may be helpful, especially for panic attacks. A starting dose of amitriptyline 10 mg can be titrated to 75 mg in the evening.

Oxygen Therapy

Oxygen therapy may be an option for some patients, particularly those with significant hypoxemia [29]. Careful individual patient assessment is required and, if the oxygen saturation is <90%, a trial of oxygen should be considered and initiated at 2 L/min for an initial duration of treatment of between 15 and 30 min. Either a mask or nasal cannulae may suit patient preference and comfort. Careful selection, assessment, and reassessment are necessary to identify those people who will benefit from oxygen therapy, and patients need to be encouraged not to become dependent on their oxygen supply, because this may severely limit their lifestyle.

Others

Other pharmacological options for breathlessness include the following [25]:

- Nebulized 0.9% sodium chloride 5 mL as required may help loosen secretions.
- Bronchodilator by inhaler, spacer, or nebulizer.
- Corticosteroids: a trial of oral dexamethasone 8–16 mg daily for lymphangitis or airway obstruction that has responded to steroids before; stop if there is no effect after a week, or reduce gradually to the lowest effective dose.
- Nebulized furosemide has been shown to reduce the sensation of breathlessness in some patient groups, although the mechanism is unclear.
- Nabilone, buspirone, bronchodilators, and methylxanthines have all been reported in the literature as successful in different patients groups, although strong evidence is lacking.

Non-pharmacological Management

The non-pharmacological management of breathlessness involves the following:

- Nurse clinics (where the intervention includes the exploration of the patient's experience of breathlessness, advice and support on managing breathlessness, and teaching breathing control and relaxation technique) experience improvement in breathlessness and performance status [30].

- Complementary therapies such as aromatherapy, hypnosis, and acupuncture may be helpful in some patients but the evidence base is weak.
- Pulmonary rehabilitation aims not only to improve pulmonary function but also to decrease pulmonary symptom burden (including breathlessness) and improve quality of life [31].

Constipation
Definition
Constipation can be defined as the passage of small hard feces infrequently and with difficulty.

Prevalence
Constipation is more common in patients with advanced cancer than in those with other terminal diseases, and many of the associated symptoms may mimic features of the underlying disease. Approximately 50% of patients admitted to specialist palliative care units report constipation, and approximately 80% of patients will require laxatives [32]. Constipation is the most frequent and most persistent adverse effect of opioid treatment. Unlike other adverse effects of opioid medication, such as nausea and vomiting, there is no, or extremely slow, tolerance build-up to the constipatory effects of opioids.

Assessment
In palliative medicine, the functional causes of constipation exceed the organic ones by far, and opioid-induced constipation is of particular importance (Figure 4.7).

A full patient history is necessary to establish the difference between current and normal pre-illness bowel patterns and to identify any psychosocial factors that may be inhibiting the patient. Aspects of the assessment should include the following:

- document previous bowel habit, current frequency, and consistency of stool,
- assess the frequency, character, and severity of any abdominal or rectal pain,
- ensure that the patient is passing flatus,

Causes of constipation			
Cancer	**Treatment**	**Debility**	**Concurrent**
Hypercalcemia	Opioids	Weakness	Hemorrhoids
Intra-abdominal or pelvic disease	Anticholinergics	Inactivity or bed rest	Anal fissure
	Anticonvulsants	Poor nutrition	Endocrine
Spinal cord compression	Antidepressants Diuretics	Insufficient fluid intake	dysfunction
Cauda equina syndrome	Aluminium salts	Inability to reach the toilet	Neurological disorders
Depression	NSAIDs	Low fiber diet	Metabolic disorders
		Confusion	Diverticulitis

Figure 4.7 Causes of constipation. (Adapted from Fallon and O'Neill [32] and Clemens and Klaschik [33])

- assess whether there is any difficulty with micturition or blockage of the urinary catheter,
- assess fluid and food intake,
- document recent medication change and laxative use,
- enquire about nausea, and
- document suspected overflow – watery fecal fluid after prolonged constipation.

Specific questions may be helpful (Figure 4.8) [34], and in opioid-induced constipation the Bowel Function Index is a simple, validated, clinician-administered, patient-reported, three-item questionnaire found to be a valuable indicator of patients' experience of symptoms [35].

With respect to the physical examination:
- check for signs of dehydration,
- check the condition of the mouth and the presence of fetid breath,
- examine the abdomen and note the quality of bowel sounds,
- check for evidence of neurological impairment (sensory or motor loss/level),
- perform rectal examination (sphincter tone, rectal content, local disease), and
- assess the patient's mental state (e.g., confusion and hypercalcemia).

Remember that the leakage of fluid feces past an impacted mass can mimic diarrhea and so, unless the history clearly suggests that diarrhea is

Taking history from patients with constipation	
Question	**Note**
When were the bowels last opened?	
What were the characteristics of the last stool?	Loose or formed, thin and ribbon-like, or small hard pellets
Was straining necessary for defecation?	
Was defecation painful?	
How characteristic of recent bowel actions was the last stool?	
What is the usual stool frequency now?	
Do you feel the need to defecate but are unable to do so?	Suggests hard stool or rectal obstruction
Is the urge to defecate largely absent?	Suggests colonic inertia
Does the stool emerge part way through a bulging anal canal outlet after significant straining?	Suggests hemorrhoids
Is there blood or mucus in the stool?	Suggests tumor obstruction, or hemorrhoids, or both

Figure 4.8 Taking history from patients with constipation. (Data from Sykes [34])

the result of acute infection, a rectal examination should be performed. On occasion, radiology may be recommended for specific patients.

General Management

The aims of management of constipation in palliative care patients are to re-establish comfortable bowel habits to the satisfaction of the patient, relieve the pain and discomfort caused by constipation, improve the patient's sense of wellbeing, restore a satisfactory level of independence in relation to bowel habits, consider individual patient preference, and prevent related GI symptoms such as nausea, vomiting, abdominal distension, and abdominal pain. General measures include the following:

- encourage a good oral fluid intake,
- high-fiber diet,
- increase physical activity,
- ensure that the patient has privacy and access to toilet facilities,
- address any reversible factors causing constipation, and
- if the current regimen is satisfactory and well tolerated, continue it but review the patient regularly and explain the importance of preventing constipation.

Not all of the above measures are possible for patients in a palliative care setting.

Pharmacological Management

Generally, a combination of a softener and a stimulant is recommended for the management of constipation in palliative care (Figure 4.9) [36].

Stimulant laxatives (e.g., senna, bisacodyl, sodium picosulfate) act directly on the myenteric nerves to evoke muscle contraction, and can reduce the absorption of water from the bowel. Their onset of action is within 6–12 h and they can produce marked colic, particularly if they are not combined with a softening agent.

Softening laxatives may be osmotic (e.g., lactulose, magnesium sulfate, polyethylene glycol), surfactant (e.g., docusate sodium, poloxamer in combination with danthron), or lubricant (e.g., liquid paraffin).

If oral laxative treatment is given the dose should be titrated upward on a daily or alternate-day basis until a bowel action is achieved. Adequate oral laxative dose titration can halve the need for rectal interventions. The occurrence of colic means that the dose of softening laxative should be increased relative to that of the stimulant, whereas the development of fecal leakage suggests a need to reduce the softening dose and perhaps increase that of the stimulant.

If fecal impaction is present, an enema or suppository may be needed; an oil or phosphate enema is indicated for impaction with hard feces, but, for a softer fecal mass, suppositories may be adequate.

Methylnaltrexone, an opioid antagonist with a restricted ability to cross the blood–brain barrier, can reduce constipation without reducing opioid analgesia [37]. It is usually given after laxatives have been tried without successful treatment of constipation.

Non-pharmacological Management

Suggested non-pharmacological approaches to the management of constipation include:

- manual evacuation,
- acupuncture/acupressure, and
- reflexology.

Pharmacological management of constipation

Prophylaxis and ongoing assessment of bowel pattern

Ongoing monitoring
- Monitor patient satisfaction with bowel pattern using checklist
- Monitor for improvements or deterioration in bowel pattern
- Monitor risk factors for constipation
- Anticipate constipating effects of pharmacological agents such as opioids
  - Prescribe laxative prophylatically

Patient education
- Encourage lifestyle changes within patient limits:
  - Increase fluid intake
  - Encourage mobility
  - Ensure privacy and comfort to allow a patient to defecate normally

Treatment

Patient complains of constipation (or in some cases if defecation <3 times/week)

Assess patient to confirm constipation → Exclude malignant intestinal obstruction

Assessment of causes

Not correctable / **Correctable**

Treatment of constipation / Treatment of causes

First-line treatment with oral laxative:
- Combination of a softer (eg, polyethylene glycol and electrolytes or lactulose) and a stimulant (eg, senna or sodium picosulphate) according to patients needs (refer to prescribing table for recommendations)

Improvement of symptoms → Continue with regimen

No improvement of symptoms

Second-line treatment:
- Rectal suppository and enema (refer to prescribing table for options)
- Consider use of a peripherally-specific opioid antagonist, eg, methylnaltrexone, if patient taking an opioid

Improvement of symptoms → Continue with regimen

No improvement of symptoms

Third-line treatment:
- Manual evacuation
- Consider use of a peripherally specific opioid antagonist, eg, methylnaltrexone, if patient taking an opioid

Improvement of symptoms → Consider next steps

Figure 4.9 Pharmacological management of constipation. (Data from Larkin et al. [36]. © 2005, reproduced with permission from John Wiley & Sons)

Cough

Definition

Cough is a primitive reflex, typically consisting of an initiating deep inspiration, glottal closure, and an explosive expiration accompanied by a sound that serves to expel mucus, sputum, fluid, and foreign bodies from the airway [38].

Prevalence

Cough has a prevalence of 23–37% in all cancers. In patients with lung cancer the prevalence is 47–86% and is moderate to severe in 17–48% of cases [39]. Cough is most common with cancers of the airways, lungs, pleura, and mediastinum, although tumors metastasizing to the thorax can also cause cough. Cough can cause significant distress by bringing symptoms such as exhaustion, sweating, incontinence, and insomnia. Furthermore, it can lead to changes in lifestyle and lowering of quality of life [40].

Assessment

In some patients it is the absence of cough that may be problematic, but for the most part it is troublesome cough that can have a negative impact on a patient's quality of life and be distressing for the family.

Some factors that decrease the effectiveness of cough in cancer patients:

- inhibitors of cough, e.g., pain, strong opioids,
- cachexia,
- steroid myopathy,
- neurological conditions causing muscle weakness,
- distended abdomen, e.g., ascites, hepatomegaly,
- vocal fold involvement, e.g., head and neck tumor, recurrent laryngeal nerve involvement,
- stiffness of major airway, e.g., endobronchial tumor, stent insertion,
- increased tenacity of mucus, e.g., dehydration, hyoscine (scopolamine), and
- decreased mucociliary clearance, e.g., smoking.

The cough can impact cancer patients in the following ways:

- sleep disturbance,
- social embarrassment, and
- interruption to communication.

Complications related to the increased thoracic pressure resulting from coughing include:

- hemodynamic changes (e.g., arrhythmias, hypotension),
- ruptured blood vessels in the nose, bronchi, or eyes (causing nosebleeds, hemoptysis, and conjunctival hemorrhage),
- urinary incontinence (stress),
- hernia,
- syncope and headache,
- pneumothorax and rib fractures,
- vomiting, and
- muscular strain.

The clinical history, physical examination (including ear, nose, and throat examination), and chest radiograph will usually define the cause of cough [41]. Other investigations (e.g., bronchoscopy) should be considered if clinically indicated.

Cough visual analog scales (VAS) are simple and commonly used in clinical studies. There are also self-completed, cough-specific, quality-of-life questionnaires including the Leicester Cough Questionnaire [42] and the Cough Specific Quality of Life Questionnaire [43], both of which are validated and include physical, psychological, and social domains. Given that subjective reports of cough are inevitably influenced by other factors such as mood, it is reasonable during assessment to combine the cough VAS with a self-report tool [44].

General Management

The general management of cough involves the following:

- identify the specific cause or underlying mechanism (Figure 4.10) [45],
- assess the effectiveness of cough, looking for factors that will diminish the cough reflex,
- assess the impact of cough on the patient's physical, social, and psychological wellbeing, and
- decide on the treatment goal and strategy (Figure 4.11) [46].

Causes of cough	
Cancer	Pulmonary parenchymal infiltration
	Lymphangitis carcinomatosis
	Intrinsic or extrinsic airway obstruction by tumor
	Pleural tumor or effusion
	Tracheo-esophageal fistula
	Multiple tumor microemboli
	Vocal fold paralysis
	Superior vena cava syndrome
Cancer therapies	Radiotherapy sequelae
	Chemotherapy induced (eg, bleomycin, cyclophosphamide)
	Chemotherapy-induced cardiomyopathy (eg, doxorubicin)
Debility	Acute coronary syndrome
	Pulmonary aspiration
	Pulmonary embolus
Other causes	Upper airway cough syndrome
	Asthma
	Gastroesophageal reflux disease
	Chronic obstructive pulmonary disease
	Bronchiectasis
	Congestive heart failure
	Angiotensin-converting enzyme inhibitor drugs
	Post-infectious cough

Figure 4.10 Causes of cough. (Data from Bonneau [45])

Pharmacological Management

Protussives

In some cases it is appropriate to encourage cough by using expectorants. Inhaled ipratropium bromide and nebulized saline are commonly used; the other options being guaifenesin or carbocisteine, which reduces the viscosity of secretions. In people with neuromuscular impairment or profound weakness, protussive agents are ineffective but mechanical cough assist devices may enhance sputum production (Figure 4.12) [47].

Antitussives

Dextromethorphan, codeine, and morphine remain the most useful and widely available oral therapies on offer. In intractable situations, nebulized local anesthetics may play a role (Figure 4.13) [41].

Specific treatment of cough in cancer patients	
Condition	**Management**
Pneumonia Sinusitis	Antibiotics
Tracheal/endobronchial tumor Lymphangitis carcinomatosis Post-irradiation lung damage Asthma Eosinophilic bronchitis PNDS	Corticosteroid
Pleural effusion Pericardial effusion	Paracentesis
Endobronchial tumor	Tumor-specific treatment: radiotherapy, laser, cryotherapy
Asthma COPD	Bronchodilators
PNDS	Antihistamine
Gastro-esophageal reflux	Proton pump inhibitor

Figure 4.11 Specific treatment of cough in cancer patients. *COPD* chronic obstructive pulmonary disorder, *PNDS* postnasal drip syndrome. (Data from Estfan and LeGrand [46])

Managing productive cough	
Tenacious sputum	Steam inhalations Nebulized saline Simple linctus Physiotherapy Active cycle breathing
Purulent sputum	Antibiotics Postural drainage Physiotherapy Cough suppression
Loose secretions but unable to cough	Positioning Antimuscarinic drugs Suction

Figure 4.12 Managing productive cough. (Data from Davis and Pervy [47])

Recommended dosages for antitussives, demulcents, and topical anesthetics

Medication	Dosage
Simple linctus	5 mL tds/qds
Dextromethorphan	10–15 mg tds/qds
Codeine	30–60 mg qds
Pholcodine	10 mL tds
Morphine (Oramorph™)	5 mg (single dose trial of Oramorph; if effective 5–10 mg slow-release morphine bd)
Diamorphine	5–10 mg CSCI q24h
Methadone linctus	Single dose 2 mg (2 mL of 1 mg/mL solution)
Dihydrocodeine	10 mg tds
Hydrocodone	5 mg bd
Inhaled cromoglicate	10 mg qds
Nebulized lidocaine*	5 mL 0.2% tds
Nebulized bupivacaine*	5 mL 0.25% tds
Prednisolone	30 mg daily for 2 weeks

Figure 4.13 Recommended dosages for antitussives, demulcents, and topical anesthetics. *CSCI* continuous subcutaneous infusion, *bd* twice daily, *qds* four times daily, *tds* three times daily. *Avoid food/drinks for at least 1 h; first dose as inpatient in case of reflex bronchospasm. (Data from Molassiotis et al. [41])

Delirium

Definition

Delirium is disturbed consciousness and inattention with cognitive impairment. It may have an acute onset and fluctuating course as a physiological consequence of disease or treatment [48].

Prevalence

Delirium is a common occurrence in the palliative care setting, which increases in prevalence with disease progression. Approximately 20–45% of admissions have delirium; 28–45% of patients develop it as inpatients, increasing to 90% in the last weeks of life [49].

Assessment

Delirium can present with a number of features and has been classified into various subtypes [50]:

- hypoactive: quiet, withdrawn, and inactive; often missed or misdiagnosed as depression,
- hyperactive: increased arousal, agitation, aggression, or hallucinations, and
- mixed pattern: features of both, fluctuates and may be worse at night.

Hypoactive and mixed delirium can be more difficult to recognize. The clinical features of delirium are as follows:
- altered conscious state,
- altered mood (excited or depressed),
- impaired short-term memory,
- impaired thinking (delusions),
- impaired judgment,
- altered perceptions (hallucinations, illusions),
- disorientation (time, person, place),
- disordered speech,
- disturbed sleep pattern (drowsy by day, insomnia at night), and
- abnormal psychomotor activity (increased or decreased).

A diagnosis of delirium depends mainly on careful clinical assessment. One should consider using the Mini-Mental State Examination or Abbreviated Mental Test (see Appendix 2).

The causes of delirium are often multifactorial and include [51]:
- drugs (including opioids, anticholinergics, steroids, benzodiazepines, antidepressants, sedatives),
- drug withdrawal (alcohol, sedatives, antidepressants, nicotine),
- dehydration, constipation, urinary retention, uncontrolled pain, and
- liver or renal impairment, electrolyte disturbance (Na^+, Ca^{2+}, glucose), infection, hypoxia, cerebral tumor, or cerebrovascular disease.

Visual impairment and deafness are risk factors. The differential diagnosis is depression or dementia (increased risk of developing delirium) (Figure 4.14) [52].

Distinguishing between delirium and dementia	
Delirium	**Dementia**
Abrupt onset	Progressive onset
Decreased level of consciousness	Level of consciousness intact, alert
Random behavior	Consistent behavior
Sleep–wake cycle changes	Minimal changes
Reversible	Irreversible

Figure 4.14 Distinguishing between delirium and dementia. (Centeno et al. [52])

General Management

Delirium in advanced cancer leads to distress in both patients and their families [53]; efforts should be made, where possible to prevent delirium (Figure 4.15) [50].

Following diagnosis of the symptom consideration should be given to identifying and managing the possible underlying cause or combination of causes (Figure 4.16) [20].

Pharmacological Management

In terminally ill patients up to 17% of patients receive an antipsychotic for agitation or psychological distress [20]. The drugs most commonly used are shown in Figures 4.17 and 4.18 [49, 54].

Terminal Delirium

In cases of terminal delirium [55]:
- review all medication and stop any non-essential drugs,
- check for opioid toxicity (drowsiness, agitation, myoclonus, hypersensitivity to touch); reduce opioid dose by a third, consider switching to another opioid if delirium persists,
- check for constipation, urinary retention, or catheter problems,
- check complete blood count (CBC) and biochemistry, including calcium,
- check for infection (urine infection in elderly people),
- if the patient is nicotine dependent, consider using replacement patches,

Interventions to prevent delirium

Clinical factor	Preventive intervention
Cognitive impairment or disorientation	Provide appropriate lighting and clear signage. A clock (consider providing a 24-hour clock in critical care) and a calendar should also be easily visible to the person at risk Re-orient the patients by explaining where they are, who they are, and what your role is Introduce cognitively stimulating activities (eg, reminiscence) Facilitate regular visits from family and friends
Dehydration or constipation	Encourage the person to drink hydrating fluids. Consider offering subcutaneous or intravenous fluids if necessary Seek advice if necessary when managing fluid balance in people with comorbidities (eg, heart failure or chronic kidney disease)
Hypoxia	Assess for hypoxia and optimize oxygen saturation if necessary
Immobility or limited mobility	Encourage the person to: • mobilize soon after surgery • walk (provide walking aids if needed; these should be accessible at all times) Encourage all people, including those unable to walk, to carry out active range-of-motion exercises
Infection	Look for and treat infection Avoid unnecessary catheterization Implement infection control procedures in line with "Infection control" (Nice Clinical Guideline 2)
Multiple medications	Carry out a medication review for people taking multiple drugs, taking into account both the type and the number of medications
Pain	Assess for pain. Look for non-verbal signs of pain, particularly in people with communication difficulties Start and review appropriate pain management in any person in whom pain is identified or suspected
Poor nutrition	Follow the advice given on nutrition in "Nutrition support in adults" (Nice Clinical Guideline 32) If the person has dentures, ensure that they fit properly
Sensory impairment	Resolve any reversible cause of the impairment (such as impacted ear wax) Ensure working hearing and visual aids are available to and used by people who need them
Sleep disturbance	Avoid nursing or medical procedures during sleeping hours, if possible Schedule medication rounds to avoid disturbing sleep Reduce noise to a minimum during sleep periods

Figure 4.15 Interventions to prevent delirium. (Data from NICE [50])

- medicate (if essential to control symptoms), and
- review regularly and withdraw medication as soon as the patient recovers.

First-Choice Treatment: Haloperidol
- Dose: 0.5–3 mg po or sc (start with a low oral dose) and repeat after 2 h, if necessary.

Causes of delirium

Direct CNS causes	Primary brain tumor, metastatic spread, seizures
Indirect causes	Metabolic encephalopathy due to organ failure, electrolyte imbalance
Medication	Steroids, opioids, anticholinergics, antiemetics, anxiolytics, antidepressants, anticonvulsants, NSAIDs
Withdrawal states	Alcohol, opioids, benzodiazepines, nicotine
Infection	Urinary tract infection, chest
Hematological abnormalities	Disseminated intravascular coagulation, bleeding (subdural hematoma)
Nutritional deficiencies Paraneoplastic syndromes	Wernicke's encephalopathy

Figure 4.16 Causes of delirium. *CNS* central nervous system, *NSAID* non-steroidal anti-inflammatory drug. (Data from Breitbart et al. [20])

Drugs used to treat delirium

Class	Drug	Approximate daily dose	Routes
Neuroleptics	Haloperidol	0.5–5 mg q2–12h	po, sc, iv, im
	Chlorpromazine	12.5–50 mg q4–12h	po, iv, im
	Levomepromazine	12.5–50 mg q4–8h	po, sc, iv
	Droperidol	0.625–2.5 mg q4–8h	im, iv
Atypical neuroleptics	Olanzapine	2.5–20 mg q12–24h	po
	Risperidone	1–3 mg q12–24h	po
Benzodiazepines	Lorazepam	0.5–2.0 mg q1–4h	po, sl, iv, im
	Midazolam	30–100 mg q24h	sc, iv
Anesthetics	Propofol	10–70 mg/hour	iv

Figure 4.17 Drugs used to treat delirium. *iv* intravenously, *im* intramuscularly, *po* orally, *sc* subcutaneously, *sl* sublingually. (Data from Breitbart et al. [20])

Mean, median, and range of sedative and antipsychotic doses in the final 48 hours of life

Drug	Mean dose (mg/day)	Median dose (mg/day)	Reported range (mg/day)
Midazolam	22–70	30–45	3–1200
Haloperidol	5	4	5–50
Chlorpromazine	21	50	13–900
Levomepromazine	64	100	25–250
Phenobarbital	–	800–1600	200–2500
Propofol	1100	500	400–9600

Figure 4.18 Mean, median, and range of sedative and antipsychotic doses in the final 48 h of life. (Data from Palliative Drugs [54])

- Maintenance treatment may be needed if the cause cannot be reversed.
- Use the lowest effective dose: 0.5–3 mg po or 2.5 mg sc od.

Second-Choice Treatment: Benzodiazepines

- Benzodiazepines do not improve cognition; they may help anxiety.
- They are used in alcohol (often at higher doses), sedative, and antidepressant withdrawal and are preferred in Parkinson's disease.
- Lorazepam should be given at a dose of 0.5–1 mg po or sl.
- Midazolam should be administered subcutaneously 2.5–5 mg 1–2 h or diazepam 5 mg po/pr q8h–q12h.

Further Sedation

In cases when further sedation is desirable and appropriate (Figure 4.17):

- Add or increase benzodiazepine (midazolam CSCI 10–30 mg/24 h in a syringe driver/pump or diazepam 5–10 mg pr q6h–q8h).
- Change haloperidol to levomepromazine 12.5–25 mg sc od/bd or as a CSCI in a syringe driver.
- Phenobarbital is one of several sedative drugs used to treat refractory agitation in the imminently dying patient. It is generally a second- or third-line treatment for patients who, for example, fail to respond to midazolam 60–120 mg/24 h and either haloperidol up to 30 mg/24 h or levomepromazine up to 200 mg/24 h.

Non-drug Delirium

In cases of non-drug delirium:

- Explain the cause and likely course to the patient, relatives, and carers.
- Address any feelings of anxiety because patients with delirium are often very frightened.
- Place the patient in a quiet area or side room; limit staff changes.
- Ensure adequate lighting, minimize noise, and provide a clock that the patient can see.
- Give the patient gentle repeated reorientation and avoid confronting deficits.
- Try to maintain normal sleep–wake cycle.
- Patients who recover recall their experiences; explain the organic cause of their behavior and symptoms.

Non-pharmacological Management

The non-pharmacological management of delirium involves the following:

- Ensure the safety of patient, family and staff.
- Reassure the family and patient of the medical nature of delirium, i.e., "Not losing your mind" or "Having a nervous breakdown."
- If this is end-stage disease, it may be necessary to tell the family that delirium is a hallmark of approaching death.
- Providing clocks, dates, time, etc., to reorient the patient has not been found to be helpful, although they may delay the onset of delirium.
- Communicate with the patient and the family. What are the goals of care and desirable outcomes? For example, sedation versus being alert but distressed.

Depression
Definition

Depression is a mental disorder that presents with depressed mood, loss of interest or pleasure, feelings of guilt or low self-worth, disturbed sleep or appetite, low energy, and poor concentration [56].

Prevalence

Depression is common in patients with life-threatening illnesses, affecting up to 75% of patients. Depression can decrease the amount of pleasure and meaning in life. It can take away hope and peace at the end of life [57]. The following are the possible presentations of depression:

- low mood, tearfulness, irritability, and distress
- withdrawal, loss of interest or pleasure in daily activities
- intractable physical symptoms or symptoms disproportionate to the degree of disease
- feelings of hopelessness, helplessness, worthlessness, or guilt
- suicidal behavior, requests for physician-assisted suicide/euthanasia, a wish to end it all, refusal of care.

Depression can also be a cause of suffering, and can increase physical pain, making the treatment of other symptoms difficult [58]. As depression is associated with an increased risk of suicide, it is important to identify depression in order to preserve quality of life.

Assessment

A number of risk factors can predispose to depression [57]:

- having a terminal illness,
- certain primary cancers (e.g., pancreatic cancer),
- comorbidities (e.g., hypothyroidism, diabetes mellitus, Alzheimer's disease, Parkinson's disease, multiple sclerosis),
- poor performance status or physical disabilities,
- poorly controlled symptoms,
- metabolic abnormalities (e.g., hypocalcemia, uremia, abnormal liver function),
- medications (e.g., amphotericin, corticosteroids, metoclopramide, cytotoxic drugs),
- radiation therapy,
- malnutrition,
- personal or family history of depression,
- younger age,
- concurrent life stresses,
- absence of social support,
- recent bereavement, and
- substance abuse.

Depression can amplify the intensity of pain and diminish one's ability to separate and say goodbye, leading to difficulties in decision-making at this critical time of one's life. It can also affect the stability of treatment preferences for life-sustaining interventions such as resuscitation. Findings indicate that depression and hopelessness are the strongest predictors of whether or not a palliative care cancer patient will have a desire for hastened death [59].

Although severe depression is generally readily recognized, the milder forms are often difficult to distinguish from emotional changes associated with everyday life. The mnemonic SADAFACES may be of assistance in a well-focused and brief interview (Figure 4.19) [60]. The Mental State Examination can be quite variable depending on the severity of the depression.

Cognitive function is intact, although in severe depression the patient may not have the interest or energy to answer, making cognitive assessment difficult [61]. The differential diagnosis of depression is as follows [62]:

Core symptoms of depression	
S	Sleep problems
A	Appetite or weight change
D	Dysphoria or bad mood
A	Anhedonia or lack of interest in pleasure
F	Fatigue
A	Agitation/psychomotor retardation
C	Concentration problems
E	Esteem problems
S	Suicidal thoughts

Figure 4.19 Core symptoms of depression. (Data from Montano [60])

- Delirium: may cause affective changes, agitation, or withdrawal; differentiating features include clouded consciousness, incoherent speech, and involuntary movements.
- Dementia: often associated with changes in mood and motivation; distinguishing features include dysphasia, poor orientation, and memory deficits.
- Ongoing physical symptoms: may cause intense distress that may be mistaken for depression, which is ameliorated when symptoms are addressed.
- Adverse drug reactions: depressed mood is a recognized side effect of many drugs, including steroids, and may be associated with opioid toxicity; depressed mood may also result from harmful alcohol/substance use or drug withdrawal (e.g., steroids and alcohol). A thorough alcohol and drug history is essential.
- Space-occupying lesion, e.g., cerebral metastases.
- Other psychiatric disorders, e.g., psychotic disorders, anxiety disorder.
- Other physical illnesses can present with depression-like symptoms, e.g., hypothyroidism.

Although low mood, weight loss, and sleep disturbance may be symptomatic of a depressive disorder, they may also be features of a normal adjustment to a life-limiting illness. Advanced disease incurs manifold losses, which the patient may grieve. It is necessary, therefore, to differentiate depression from normal grief. The inability to differentiate the symptoms of each is one of the reasons for the under-detection of depression in palliative care [63]. Numerous screening tools have been utilized in an effort to improve the identification of depression in palliative care, including the HADS [18] (see Appendix 2).

General Management
The general management of depression involves identifying and managing the possible underlying cause or combination of causes.

Pharmacological Management
There is limited evidence for the effectiveness of pharmacological interventions in treatment of depression in cancer patients. When a drug is prescribed, therefore, the following should be taken into account:
- the presence of additional physical health disorders
- the adverse effects of prescribed drug which may impact on the underlying physical disease
- interactions with other medications.

Antidepressants
Antidepressants are the mainstay of pharmacological treatment in depression (Figure 4.20) [20] and TCAs and the SSRIs are the two groups commonly used in the palliative care population. Although amitriptyline is widely available and inexpensive, and has equal or better efficacy than other antidepressants, it causes more undesirable effects.

Antidepressants take time to work, particularly when slow-dose escalation is necessary with TCAs, the median response time for depression in older patients is said to be 2–3 months, whereas mirtazapine and venlafaxine appear to be faster acting.

When switching from one antidepressant to another, prescribers should be aware of the need for gradual and modest incremental increases of dose, interactions between antidepressants, and the risk of serotonin toxicity when combinations of serotonergic antidepressants are prescribed. Discontinuation of antidepressants should be done gradually if the patient has been taking them for more than 8 weeks to prevent withdrawal symptoms.

Antidepressant medication used in patients with advanced disease

Class	Drug	Approximate daily oral dose (mg)
TCAs	Amitriptyline	10–150
	Doxepin	12.5–150
	Imipramine	12.5–150
	Desipramine	12.5–150
	Nortriptyline	12–125
	Clomipramine	10–150
SSRIs	Fluoxetine	20–160
	Sertraline	50–200
	Paroxetine	10–60
	Citalopram	10–60
	Escitalopram	10–40
	Fluvoxamine	50–300
Serotonin–norepinephrine reuptake inhibitor	Venlafaxine	75–225
Norepinephrine and dopamine reuptake blockers	Mirtazepine	15–60
Psychostimulants	Dexamfetamine	2.5–2.0 bd
	Methylphenidate	2.5–2.0 bd
	Modafinil	50–400
MAOIs	Isocarboxazid	20–40
	Phenelzine	30–60
	Tranylcypromine	20–40
	Moclobemide	100–600
Benzodiazepines	Alprazolam	0.25–2.0 tds
Lithium carbonate		600–1200

Figure 4.20 Antidepressant medication used in patients with advanced disease. *bd* twice daily, *tds* three times daily, *MAOI* monoamine oxidase inhibitor, *SSRI* selective serotonin reuptake inhibitor, *TCAs* tricyclic antidepressants. (Data from Breitbart et al. [20])

Psychostimulants have been suggested as a rapid-onset treatment of depression, especially suitable to those with a very short life expectancy. There are reports that dexamphetamine and methylphenidate can be effective within hours or days. However, a systematic review of psychostimulants for treatment of depression in any context found insufficient evidence to recommend them [64].

Lithium is widely used in psychiatric practice as a mood stabilizer. It has a narrow therapeutic index and the co-prescription of non-steroidal anti-inflammatory drugs (NSAIDs) can inhibit the renal excretion of lithium and increase plasma concentrations with increased risk of severe toxicity.

Non-pharmacological Management

Psychological interventions are increasingly seen as part of a comprehensive package of psychosocial input for patients with advanced cancer. For people with persistent depressive symptoms or mild-to-moderate depression, the following interventions may be considered, guided by the person's preference.

Strategies include [64]:

- cognitive–behavioral therapy,
- couples therapy, and
- supportive expressive group therapy.

Complementary Therapies

Aromatherapy massage has been shown to be effective for depression in patients with advanced cancer [65].

Consider collaborative care with the mental health services for patients with moderate-to-severe depression with associated functional impairment whose depression has not responded to initial high-intensity psychological interventions, pharmacological treatment, or a combination of psychological and pharmacological interventions [66].

Diarrhea
Definition

Diarrhea is the passage of frequent loose stools with urgency.

Prevalence

In advanced cancer patients, the prevalence of diarrhea is approximately 7–10% of patients admitted to a hospice and 6% of similar patients in hospital [34]. Diarrhea is an embarrassing and debilitating problem, and potential causes include overuse of laxatives, infective agents, antibiotics,

Causes of diarrhea in palliative medicine	
Drugs	Laxatives, antacids, antibiotics, chemotherapy agents (eg, 5-flurouracil, irinotecan), iron salts
Radiation	
Obstruction	Malignant, fecal, narcotic bowel syndrome
Malabsorption	Pancreatic carcinoma, gastrectomy, ileal resection, colectomy
Tumor	Colonic or rectal cancer, pancreatic islet cell tumors, carcinoid tumors
Concurrent disease	Diabetes mellitus, hyperthyroidism, inflammatory bowel disease, irritable bowel syndrome
Diet	Bran, fruit, hot spices, alcohol

Figure 4.21 Causes of diarrhea in palliative medicine. (Data from Sykes [34])

chemotherapy, radiotherapy, surgery, malnutrition, paraneoplastic disorders, neuroendocrine tumors, and neoplastic bowel infiltration [67].

Assessment

The causes of diarrhea in palliative care patients can be multifactorial (Figure 4.21) [34]. It can present as acute or chronic and assessment will require the usual process including the following:

- medical history,
- physical examination,
- stool culture,
- blood tests,
- fasting tests,
- radiology,
- sigmoidoscopy, and
- colonoscopy.

Watery diarrhea may be a sign of fecal impaction.

General Management

Review diet, medications, laxatives, procedures, timing of movements in relation to ingestion of food or liquids, and a description of and quantity and quality of stool. Patients at the end of life are also at risk of developing the same diarrheal illnesses that occur every day in the general population, which require specific management (Figure 4.22) [34].

Specific treatments for diarrhea	
Fat malabsorption	Pancreatin (may be more effective if H2-receptor antagonist given before meals
Chologenic diarrhea	Cholestyramine 4–12 g tds
Radiation-induced diarrhea	Aspirin, cholestyramine 4–12 g tds
Zollinger–Ellison syndrome	H2-receptor antagonist, eg, ranitidine initially 150 mg tds
Carcinoid syndrome	Cyproheptadine, initially 12 mg/day, methylsergide 12–20 mg/day
Pseudomembranous colitis	Vancomycin 125 mg qds, metronidazole 400 mg tds
Ulcerative colitis	Mesalazine 1.2–2.4 g/day, corticosteroids

Figure 4.22 Specific treatments for diarrhea. (Data from Sykes [34])

Pharmacological Management

Antimotility Drugs

Antimotility drugs relieve the symptoms of acute diarrhea and are used in the management of uncomplicated acute diarrhea in adults. Fluid and electrolyte replacement may be necessary in case of dehydration [20].

In acute diarrhea, loperamide 4 mg is initially administered followed by 2 mg after each loose stool for up to 5 days. The usual dose is 6–8 mg/day up to a maximum of 16 mg/day. In chronic diarrhea in adults, loperamide is administered initially, 4–8 mg/day in divided doses, and is subsequently adjusted according to response and given in two divided doses for maintenance, up to a maximum of 16 mg/day. When chronic diarrhea persists, codeine phosphate and morphine can also be used and titrated to effect [20].

Antimuscarinics

Antimuscarinics, which are used for the management of irritable bowel syndrome and diverticular disease, are occasionally of value in treating abdominal cramp associated with diarrhea. They include the tertiary amines atropine sulfate and dicycloverine hydrochloride, and the quaternary ammonium compounds propantheline bromide and hyoscine (scopolamine) butylbromide [20].

Hyoscine (scopolamine) butylbromide (Buscopan®) should be started at 20 mg qds, noting that oral absorption is poor. Sublingual hyoscine (scopolamine) preparations may be used as an alternative. Dicyclomine hydrochloride (Merbentyl) should be given at a dose of 10–20 mg tds.

Adsorbents

Adsorbents such as kaolin can be of help in chronic diarrhea. Bulk-forming drugs, such as ispaghula, methylcellulose, and sterculia, are useful in controlling diarrhea associated with diverticular disease. Available formulations include kaolin oral suspension, light kaolin or light kaolin (natural) 20%, light magnesium carbonate 5%, and sodium bicarbonate 5% in a suitable vehicle with a peppermint flavor [7]. The recommended dose is 10–20 mL q4h. A kaolin and morphine oral suspension is also available.

Somatostatin Analog

Octreotide is effective with profuse secretory diarrhea and those with high effluent volume from a stoma. It may be given via CSCI. The starting dose is 50–500 µg/day, and daily doses as high as 1,500 µg have been used. Once improvement is achieved the dose is reduced to the lowest dose that maintains symptom control.

Non-pharmacological Management

Ensure adequate hydration and encourage sips of clear liquids. Intravenous hydration should be considered in cases of severe dehydration. Simple carbohydrates, toast, or crackers will add back small amounts of electrolytes and glucose. Milk and other lactose-containing products should be avoided.

Dry Mouth
Definition

Dry mouth (or xerostomia) is a subjective sensation of dryness of the mouth.

Prevalence

The problem of dry mouth is common in advanced cancer, affecting up to 70% of patients [68]. Dry mouth most commonly results from a reduction in the amount of saliva secreted, although a change in the composition of saliva can also lead to the sensation. The most common cause of dry mouth in patients with cancer is drug treatment including analgesics, adjuvant analgesics, and antiemetics (Figure 4.23) [69].

Causes of dry mouth	
Diseases of, or damage to, salivary glands	
Cancer-related	Tumor infiltration
Treatment-related	Surgery, radiotherapy, chemotherapy
Not related to cancer	Sjögren's syndrome
Damage to, or interference with, salivary gland nerve supply	
Cancer-related	Tumor infiltration
Treatment-related	Surgery, radiotherapy, drugs
Not related to cancer	Dementia
Interference with productive capacity of salivary glands	
Drugs	
Dehydration	
Malnutrition	
Other causes	
Drugs	
Decreased oral intake	
Decreased mastication	
Anxiety	
Depression	

Figure 4.23 Causes of dry mouth. (Data from Davies [69])

Assessment

Dry mouth may be associated with a number of local signs and symptoms and can have a profound negative impact on quality of life. The lack of salivary secretions impacts the ability to eat, sleep, speak, and swallow. A dry mouth can lead to changes in taste, which in turn decreases appetite and can lead to subsequent weight loss and malnutrition [70]. Patients with dry mouth have difficulty with dry or thick food, and their meals are frequently interrupted with sips of fluid to aid chewing and swallowing. Sleep can be affected because rest is frequently interrupted due to oral dryness. The patient may wake frequently with the tongue adhered to the hard palate and needing to expectorate frequently or manually remove thick saliva [71].

In cases of chronic dry mouth, patients may present with recurrent oral infections, the deterioration or atrophy of the oral epithelium, and painful excoriation and ulceration. Candida infection and other oral infections common to the tongue or buccal mucosa are widely seen. Dental manifestations such as dental caries and periodontal disease also commonly occur.

General Management

If possible the underlying cause should be treated, including a review of the medication. Patients may benefit from the advice of a dentist or oral hygienist and comprehensive mouth care. Management of dry mouth is as follows [72]:

- oral hygiene every 2 h,
- humidified air,
- suck ice cubes, vitamin C tablets, frozen tonic water,
- chew sugar-free chewing gum, citrus sweets, pineapple pieces,
- artificial saliva and oral lubricants,
- avoid alcohol including mouth rinses that contain alcohol,
- pilocarpine,
- review dose or stop drugs contributing to dry mouth, and
- correct dehydration.

Pharmacological Management

Saliva substitutes can provide useful relief of dry mouth. A properly balanced artificial saliva should have a neutral pH and contain electrolytes that correspond approximately to the composition of saliva. For maximum effect, artificial salivas or topical saliva stimulants need to be taken every 30–60 min, and before and during meals.

Saliva stimulants can increase the production of normal saliva and so ameliorate both the dry mouth and the other complications of hyposalivation. Pilocarpine tablets are licensed for the treatment of xerostomia after irradiation for head and neck cancer, provided that patients have some residual salivary gland function. A dose of 5 mg tds should be given with or immediately after meals (the last dose is always given with the evening meal). If the dose is tolerated, but the response is insufficient after 4 weeks, it may be increased to a maximum of 30 mg/day in divided doses. The maximum therapeutic effect usually occurs within 4–8 weeks. Pilocarpine should be discontinued if there is no improvement after 2–3 months [7]. Bethanecol is an alternative to pilocarpine, and the usual dose is 10–25 mg tds/qds.

Non-pharmacological Management

Options for the non-pharmacological management of dry mouth include:

- sipping semi-frozen drinks,

- sucking ice cubes,
- chewing pineapple pieces,
- sugar-free chewing gum, and
- acupuncture.

Dysphagia

Definition

Dysphagia refers either to the difficulty someone may have with initiating a swallow or to the sensation that foods and/or liquids are somehow hindered in their passage from the mouth to the stomach [73].

Prevalence

The prevalence of dysphagia in palliative care ranges from 9% to 55% depending on the population group studied. Patients with head and neck cancers, for example, have a higher prevalence.

Assessment

There are multiple causes of dysphagia that can occur alone or in combination (Figure 4.24) [74].

A number of factors may compromise swallowing [75]:

- old age,
- lack of time to eat,
- missing teeth,
- poor environment,
- uninteresting, tepid food,
- insufficient staff to help,
- drowsiness,

Causes of dysphagia	
Disease	Xerostomia, mucosal infection, mucositis, surgery, dentition, post-radiation fibrosis, dystonic reactions, pharyngeal pathology, esophageal pathology, intraluminal obstruction, external compression, drugs altering esophageal tone, anxiety
Neurological	Upper motor neuron damage, lower motor neuron damage, direct nerve damage, cerebellar damage, paraneoplastic, neuromuscular
Other	Concurrent diseases, drowsiness, pain, extreme weakness, depression, hypercalcemia

Figure 4.24 Causes of dysphagia. (Data from Swann and Edmonds [74])

- low mood, and
- dry mouth.

The following are the key features to consider in the medical history:
- location,
- types of foods and/or liquids,
- progressive or intermittent, and
- duration of symptoms.

Oropharyngeal Dysphagia

In oropharyngeal dysphagia, patients have difficulty initiating a swallow, and they usually identify the cervical area as the area presenting a problem. Frequent accompanying symptoms include nasal regurgitation, coughing, nasal speech, diminished cough reflex, choking, and halitosis [73].

Esophageal Dysphagia

Esophageal dysphagia occurs equally with solids and liquids. It often involves an esophageal motility problem when it may be associated with chest pain. Dysphagia that occurs only with solids suggests the possibility of mechanical obstruction. If progressive, consider particularly peptic stricture or carcinoma [73]. Investigations include the following:
- chest radiograph,
- barium swallow,
- upper GI endoscopy,
- computed tomography (CT) scan,
- endoscopic ultrasonography,
- test swallow, and
- speech and language therapy assessment.

General Management

General management of dysphagia involves the following [74]:
- education and explanation to the patient and carers,
- comprehensive and regular mouth care,
- dental assessment,
- frequent small meals,

Pharmacological treatments for dysphagia	
Esophageal candidiasis	Fluconazole 50 mg/day
Viral esophageal ulceration	Aciclovir 200–800 mg five times a day
Esophageal mucositis	Patient-controlled analgesia Sucralfate 10 mL 2–4 hours Maalox 5–10 mL qds
Peritumoral edema	Dexamethasone 16 mg sc
Tumor bleeding	Tranexamic acid 1 g qds
Sialorrhea	Amitriptyline 10 mg at night Hyoscine (scopolamine) hydrobromide transdermal patch Glycopyrrollate/hyoscine (scopolamine) hydrobromide CSCI Salivary gland irradiation

Figure 4.25 Pharmacological treatments for dysphagia. *CSCI* continuous subcutaneous infusion, *qds* four times daily, *sc* subcutaneously. (Data from Swann and Edmonds [74])

- soft diet,
- add calories to food or add high-calorie supplements,
- thickened fluids to aid swallowing, and
- review medication and discontinue drugs that may exacerbate swallowing difficulties.

Pharmacological Management

Specific reversible causes of dysphagia may be amenable to pharmacological management (Figure 4.25) [74].

Non-pharmacological Management

Specific palliative procedures may be appropriate, depending on the history, previous therapy and response, the patient's performance status, and preferences, including endoscopic dilation of esophageal obstruction, esophageal intubation, endoscopic laser therapy, external beam radiotherapy, brachytherapy, chemotherapy, and non-oral feeding. Indications and contraindication for choosing non-oral feeding route are shown in Figure 4.26 [75].

Halitosis
Definition

Halitosis is an offensive odor from the mouth, pharynx, nose, or sinus.

Indications and contraindication for choosing non-oral feeding route

All routes	Intravenous	Nasogastric tube	Subcutaneous	Gastrostomy
Indications				
Oral and pharyngeal transit time >10 seconds	Complete pharyngeal or esophageal obstruction	Medium-term use (1–3 weeks)	Medium-term use (1–3 weeks)	Long-term use (4 weeks or more)
Failure to modify swallowing technique during treatment to improve muscle control	Short-term use for hydration Anatomical or functional bowel loss		Hyperactive delirium due to dehydration	
Nutritional support for surgery or chemotherapy				
Contraindications				
Rapid deterioration Cachexia	Hyperactive delirium	Hyperactive delirium	Extensive skin disease	Hyperactive delirium
Psychological need of staff or family to provide active treatment	Presence of sepsis Limited or no access to biochemical monitoring Limited or no access to a parenteral nutrition team Superior vena cava obstruction	Nasal pharyngeal or esophageal obstruction Cosmetic appearance Long-term use (4 weeks or more)		Intra-abdominal disease

Figure 4.26 Indications and contraindication for choosing non-oral feeding route. (Data from Regnard [75])

Prevalence

The reported prevalence of halitosis has been as high as 50% [76]. Approximately 80–90% of objective halitosis is caused by oral conditions [77].

Assessment

Halitosis may be classified as genuine halitosis, pseudo-halitosis, and halitophobia. Genuine halitosis can be divided into physiological and pathological halitosis. If oral malodor does not exist but the patient

Causes of halitosis	
Diseases of the oral cavity	Poor hygiene Dental plaque, decay, cancer, bleeding gums Tongue coating Dry mouth Acute necrotizing gingivitis Oral malignancy
Diseases of the respiratory tract	Infection of nose, tongue, nasal sinuses, pharynx, lungs Tonsillar abscess, necrotic ulcers Chronic rhinitis and rhinopharyngitis Pharyngeal–laryngeal cancer with superinfection Bronchiectasis, lung abscess Abscess forming lung cancer
Diseases of the digestive tract	Esophageal diverticula, hiatus hernia, gastric stasis Gastroesophageal reflux disease Pyloric stenosis or duodenal obstruction Altered secretion or bile composition, colon stasis
Metabolic failure	Diabetic ketoacidosis Renal failure Hepatic failure
Drugs	Causing dry mouth and/or taste alteration Cytotoxic drugs causing oral complications Dimethyl sulfoxide, antibiotics Nitrites and nitrates, chloral hydrate or iodine-based drugs
Foods	Garlic, onions, leeks, radishes
Alcohol, tobacco	

Figure 4.27 Causes of halitosis

believes that it does, the diagnosis would be pseudo-halitosis. If, after treatment for either genuine or pseudo-halitosis, the patient still believes that he or she has halitosis, the diagnosis would be halitophobia [78].

Physiological halitosis is the most common type and is not caused by underlying disease. Pathological halitosis usually results from diseases of the oral cavity, but may be associated with diseases of the respiratory or GI tract, or a systemic metabolic problem (Figure 4.27) [72].

The clinical assessment of halitosis is usually subjective and based on smelling the exhaled air of the nose and mouth; in some cases patients perceive halitosis but it cannot be detected by others. Odor detectable from the mouth alone is likely to be of oral or pharyngeal origin whereas odor detectable form the nose alone is likely to originate from the nose or sinuses. Odors

Nature of halitosis	
Putrefied	Anerobic infection
Sweet/sickly	Pseudomonas infection
Ammonia	Renal failure
Sweet, fecal (fetor hepaticus)	Hepatic failure
Sweet acetone	Diabetic ketoacidosis

Figure 4.28 Nature of halitosis

arising from both nose and mouth are likely to have a systemic cause [76]. The nature of the halitosis may be evident from the odor (Figure 4.28).

General Management

Management requires establishing the presence of true halitosis and assessing its severity. When halitosis is not due to the underlying disease, the following is recommended [72]:

- regular oral hygiene, including tongue cleaning and good care of dentures,
- regular use of antimicrobial toothpastes and mouthwashes,
- denture care,
- dietary advice, and reduce alcohol intake and smoking,
- treatment of non-oral causes, and
- review drug regimen.

Where halitosis is due to underlying disease of the oral cavity, diseases of the respiratory or GI tract, or a systemic problem, treatment is aimed at the underlying condition.

Pharmacological Management
Mouthwash

Regular use of a gargle or mouthwash containing an antimicrobial agent may reduce breath odor; use saliva stimulants or substitutes if the mouth is very dry:

- Rinse mouth with 10 mL chlorhexidine gluconate 0.2% for approximately 1 min bd.
- Spray AS Saliva Orthana® bd/tds on to oral and pharyngeal mucosa, when required.

- Apply Biotène® Oral Balance to the gums and tongue as required.
- Spray Glandosane® aerosol spray on to the oral and pharyngeal mucosa when required.
- Pilocarpine 5 mg tds.
- Bethanecol 10–25 mg tds/qds.

Antimicrobial Therapy

Halitosis resulting from infection may respond to antimicrobial therapy. Metronidazole can be used in cases of anerobic infections (usually treated for 7 and 10–14 days in *Clostridium difficile* infection), by mouth, either 800 mg initially then 400 mg tds or 500 mg tds; for acute oral infections, by mouth, 200 mg tds for 3–7 days.

Non-pharmacological Management

Options for the non-pharmacological management of halitosis include the following [79]:
- masking agents such as mints and cosmetic sprays, and
- natural products such as black tea and various herbs.

Hiccups
Definition

Hiccups are a repeated, involuntary, spasmodic contraction of the diaphragm and inspiratory muscles followed by sudden closure of the glottis [80].

Prevalence

In a general palliative care population approximately 2% of patients have hiccups [1]. In patients with advanced cancer, gastric distension is considered the most likely cause of this symptom. In patients with advanced cancer, hiccups lasting more than 48 h are not uncommon, and can be very distressing. The consequences of persistent hiccups are [81]:
- disturbed sleep,
- reduced oral intake,
- interrupted speech,
- pain,
- reflux esophagitis,

Causes of persistent hiccups	
Iatrogenic	Surgical procedures: abdominal or thoracic operations, neck extension during intubation Drugs, eg, diazepam, dexamethasone, methylprednisolone, midazolam, megestrol acetate, morphine
Intrathoracic	Esophageal disorders (eg, reflux, obstruction, cancer), hiatus hernia, lung cancer, mediastinal tumor, respiratory infection, myocardial infarction, thoracic aneurysm
Intra-abdominal	Gastric distension, gastrointestinal bleeding, gastric cancer, pancreatic cancer, hepatomegaly, ascites, bowel obstruction
CNS	Intracranial tumor, encephalitis, head injury, cerebral vascular disease
Metabolic	Renal failure, hyponatremia, hypocalcemia, hypocapnia, sepsis
Psychogenic	Hysteria, personality disorder, grief reaction

Figure 4.29 Causes of persistent hiccups. *CNS* central nervous system. (Data from Perdue and Lloyd [81])

- anxiety, fatigue, depression, and
- wound dehiscence (if recent abdominal or thoracic surgery).

Assessment

The causes of hiccups in patients with advanced cancer may be multifactorial (Figure 4.29) [81]. Hiccups may be mild and intermittent or continuous and severe, thereby causing severe distress. An assessment of the impact of hiccups on patients is therefore important before proceeding to management.

General Management

General management of hiccups involves the following:
- treatment of reversible factors,
- hiccups often stop spontaneously,
- treatment required only if hiccups are persistent, and
- try simple physical maneuvers initially and those that worked in the past.

Pharmacological Management

Prokinetic

The prokinetic pharmacological management of hiccups involves the following [82, 83]:
- oral domperidone or metoclopramide 10–20 mg tds,
- treat any gastroesophageal reflux with a PPI, and

- dexamethasone 4–8 mg po in the morning may reduce compression/irritation if the patient has a hepatic or cerebral tumor. Stop if there is no benefit after a week.

Other Options

Other pharmacological options include the following [75]:

- baclofen 5–20 mg tds po,
- gabapentin 300–600 mg q8h po,
- nifedipine 10–20 mg tds po/sl,
- haloperidol 1.5–3 mg po at night,
- methylphenidate 10 mg po, and
- midazolam 10–30 mg/24 h CSCI, reducing the dose as the patient improves.

Non-pharmacological Management

Non-pharmacological approaches to the management of hiccup include the following [75]:

- sipping iced water or swallowing crushed ice,
- breathing into a paper bag, particularly if the patient is hyperventilating,
- interrupting normal breathing, e.g., holding breath,
- rubbing the soft palate with a swab to stimulate the nasopharynx,
- stimulating the pharynx with an oral catheter,
- nebulized saline, and
- acupuncture.

Insomnia
Definition

Insomnia is a subjective sensation of poor quality sleep.

Prevalence

Insomnia is a common symptom with a reported prevalence of 40% in cancer patients [84]. It is more common in women, elderly people, and those with a previous history of insomnia or a coexisting psychiatric illness [85]. The presence of insomnia can lead to fatigue, cognitive impairment, mood disturbance, and physical symptoms such as headache [86].

Factors contributing to insomnia

Factor	Notes
Depression	Major depressive illness related to loss, chronic pain, effects of tumor on CNS, metabolic/endocrine disturbance
Anxiety	Adjustment disorder or generalized anxiety related to fears of illness, procedures, pain or death; medication; direct effects on CNS
Cognitive impairment	Delirium secondary to medication, metabolic disorders, direct involvement of CNS
Fever	With or without sweats, chills
Pain	Related to direct tumor effects, diagnostic or treatment interventions, non-specific causes
Nausea and vomiting	Associated with chemotherapy, medications, or primary gastrointestinal disturbance
Respiratory distress	Breathlessness due to hypoxia and/or anxiety, obstructive sleep apnea, pleuritic pain
Medication	Stimulants, bronchodilators, steroids, antihypertensives, antidepressants; withdrawal or rebound from sedative hypnotics or analgesics
Psychophysiological	Caused by conditional arousal response, negative expectations, and poor sleep habits
Sleep–wake schedule	Associated with disruption of normal schedule, excessive time in bed or napping, disturbed nocturnal sleep
Environmental	Light, noise, frequent interruptions, lack of privacy
Restless leg syndrome	Secondary or peripheral neuropathy, Parkinson's disease, iron deficiency, antidepressant medication, caffeinism, sedative hypnotic withdrawal, anemia, uremia, leukemia

Figure 4.30 Factors contributing to insomnia. *CNS* central nervous system. (Data from Sateia and Byock [87])

Assessment

Insomnia is a symptom rather than a diagnosis, and multiple factors may contribute (Figure 4.30) [87]. Physical factors related to the disease that may be preventing or disturbing sleep require assessment and management [88].

General Management

Sleep hygiene involves a series of relatively simple measures that can promote good sleep [87]:

- Maintain as regular a sleep–wake schedule as possible, particularly with respect to the hour of morning waking.
- Avoid unnecessary time in bed during the day; for bedbound patients, prompt as much cognitive and physical stimulation during daytime hours as conditions permit.

- Nap only as necessary, and avoid napping in late afternoon and evening whenever possible.
- Keep as active a daytime schedule as possible; this should include social contacts and, when able, light exercise.
- Minimize nighttime sleep interruptions due to medication, noise, or other environmental factors.
- Avoid lying in bed for prolonged periods at night in an alert and frustrated or tense state; read or engage in other relaxing activity.
- Remove unpleasant conditioned stimuli, such as clocks, from sight and sound.
- Identify problems and concerns of the day before tryingto sleep and address these issues with an active problem-solving approach.
- Avoid stimulating medication and other substances, particularly in the hours before bedtime.
- Maintain adequate pain relief through the night, preferably with modified-release (MR) analgesics.
- Use sleep medication as indicated after proper evaluation of the sleep problem, and avoid overusage.

Pharmacological Management

Short-acting hypnotics are preferable in patients with sleep-onset insomnia, when sedation the following day is undesirable, or when prescribing for elderly patients. Long-acting hypnotics are indicated in patients with poor sleep maintenance (e.g., early morning waking) that causes daytime effects, when an anxiolytic effect is needed during the day, or when sedation the following day is acceptable. Hypnotics and anxiolytics may impair judgment and increase reaction time, and so affect the ability to drive or operate machinery. They increase the effects of alcohol. Moreover, the hangover effects of a night dose may impair driving on the following day [7].

Benzodiazepines are the most popular class of medication for the management of insomnia (Figure 4.31). Examples of benzodiazepines used as hypnotics include nitrazepam and flurazepam which have a pro-longed action and may give rise to residual effects on the following day; repeated doses tend to be cumulative. Loprazolam, lormetazepam, and temazepam act for a shorter time and they have little or no hangover effect. Withdrawal phenomena are more common with the short-acting

Pharmacological management of insomnia	
Drug	**Usual dose**
Temazepam	10–20 mg at night, exceptional circumstances 30–40 mg
Nitrazepam	5–10 mg at night
Flurazepam	15–30 mg at night
Loprazolam	1 mg at night, increased to 1.5 or 2 mg prn
Lormetazepam	0.5–1.5 mg at night
Zaleplon	10 mg at night or after going to bed if difficulty falling asleep
Zolpidem	10 mg at night
Zopiclone	3.75–7.5 mg at night

Figure 4.31 Pharmacological management of insomnia. (Data from Palliative Drugs [54])

benzodiazepines. If insomnia is associated with daytime anxiety then the use of a long-acting benzodiazepine anxiolytic such as diazepam given as a single dose at night may effectively treat both symptoms [7].

The following hypnotics can be used:

- Zaleplon, zolpidem, and zopiclone are non-benzodiazepine hypnotics, but they act in a similar way. Zolpidem and zopiclone have a short duration of action, and zaleplon is very short acting.
- Clomethiazole (Heminevrin®) may be a useful hypnotic for elderly patients because of its freedom from hangover. The recommended dose is 1–2 caps at night.
- Chloral hydrate and derivatives were formerly popular hypnotics for children. There is no convincing evidence that they are particularly useful in elderly people and their role as hypnotics is now very limited.
- Although some antihistamines such as promethazine are on sale to the public for occasional insomnia, their prolonged duration of action can often cause drowsiness the following day. The sedative effect of antihistamines may diminish after a few days of continued treatment.
- Melatonin is a pineal hormone; it is licensed for the short-term treatment of insomnia in adults age >55 years. The recommended dose is 2 mg od 1–2 h before bedtime for 3 weeks.

Non-pharmacological Management
Complementary Therapies

Acupuncture, hypnotherapy, aromatherapy, and reflexology have all been reported as beneficial in the management of insomnia; however, a systematic review of the literature found only evidentiary support in the treatment of chronic insomnia for acupressure, t'ai chi, yoga, mixed evidence for acupuncture and L-tryptophan, and weak and unsupportive evidence for herbal medicines such as valerian [89].

Cognitive–Behavioral Therapy
This can help through considering the situation (insomnia) and the associated thoughts, emotions, physical feelings, and actions. It is not a quick fix but is free from the adverse effects seen with pharmacological management and should be considered in palliative care patients [90].

Itch
Definition
Itch is defined as an irritating skin sensation causing a desire to scratch.

Prevalence
Itch (pruritus) is prevalent in 5–12% of palliative care patients [91]. It may be associated with any malignancy, although hematological malignancies are commonly associated with itch. Severe itch in Hodgkin's disease can predict a poor prognosis. Itch may also be a sign of biliary obstruction from either primary or secondary tumor, although there is no clear association between the level of bilirubin and severity of itch [92].

Assessment
Itch can cause discomfort, frustration, poor sleep, anxiety, and depression [93] and persistent scratching leads to skin damage (i.e., excoriation and thickening). Itch may be classified as either primary or secondary. Primary or idiopathic itch is identified in most patients where dermatological disease has been excluded (Figure 4.32) [93]. It is often fairly limited in extent and intensity.

Secondary itch may be localized or due to systemic disease (Figure 4.33) [94].

General Management
As itch is often associated with dry skin, an emollient is usually tried first. If reversible causes exist (e.g., malignant obstruction of the bile duct), these should be addressed [93]:

Evaluation of itch without obvious cause

History	Periodicity (day or night, intermittent or continuous), nature (burning, prickling, insects crawling), location, provoking factors (activity, cold, sunlight, water), drugs (opioids, hypersensitivity), atopic history, travel history
Examination	Dry skin, scabies, icteric conjunctivae, weight loss, mental state
Laboratory investigations	CBC, erythrocyte sedimentation rate, plasma creatinine, LFTs, thyroid function tests, fasting plasma glucose, fecal analysis for parasitic ova
Other investigations	Chest radiograph, abdominal ultrasonography, skin biopsy

Figure 4.32 **Evaluation of itch without obvious cause**. *CBC* complete blood count, *LFTs* liver function tests. (Data from Twycross and Greaves [93])

Potential causes of itch in a palliative care setting

Skin diseases	Eczema, bullous pemphigoid, contact dermatitis, cutaneous T lymphoma, dermatitis herpetiformis, drugs, folliculitis, lichen planus, pityriasis rosea, pruritus ani and vulvae, psoriasis, scabies, sunburn, systemic parasitic infection, urticaria
Biliary and hepatic	Biliary atresia, primary biliary cirrhosis, sclerosing cholangitis, extrabiliary obstruction, drug-induced cholestasis
Chronic renal failure	
Drugs	Opioids, amfetamines, aspirin subclinical drug sensitivity
Endocrine	Diabetes insipidus, diabetes mellitus, parathyroid disease, hypothyroidism, hyperthyroidism
Hemopoietic	Hodgkin's and non-Hodgkin's lymphoma, cutaneous T lymphoma, systemic mastocytosis, multiple myeloma, polycythemia rubra vera, iron deficiency anemia
Infection	Syphilis, parasitic, HIV, fungal
Malignancy	Breast cancer, stomach cancer, lung cancer, carcinoid syndrome
Neurological	Stroke, multiple sclerosis, tabes dorsalis, brain abscess/tumors, psychosis

Figure 4.33 **Potential causes of itch in a palliative care setting**. (Data from Pittelkow and Loprinzi [94])

- cutting nails to avoid trauma,
- use an emollient or aqueous cream frequently as a moisturizer,
- add an emollient to bath water and use aqueous cream as a soap substitute,
- exclude dermatoses, especially scabies,

- biliary stenting: may relieve the symptoms of cholestatic jaundice, and
- review medication to exclude a drug reaction (e.g., opioid switch if morphine induced).

Pharmacological Management

No broad-spectrum drug treatment exists, although several topical and systemic treatments are available that suppress itching in certain clinical settings.

Topical Therapy

- Aqueous cream (1% menthol can be added).
- Crotamiton 10% cream (Eurax®) or capsaicin (0.025%) cream for localized itch.
- A topical corticosteroid may be used once daily for 2–3 days if the area is inflamed but not infected.

Systemic Therapy

- Antihistamine (stop if no benefit seen after a few days).
- Use a sedating antihistamine if poor sleep is a problem (e.g., chlorphenamine, hydroxyzine).
- Some non-sedating antihistamines can have an antipruritic effect (e.g., loratadine, cetirizine).
- An antidepressant can help if the patient has associated anxiety or depression.
- Ondansetron 4 mg bd po increased to 8 mg bd if required.
- Paroxetine 20 mg od.
- Cimetidine 400 mg bd for itch in lymphoma or polycythemia.

Non-pharmacological Management

Non-pharmacological management of itch involves the following:

- patients may benefit from keeping cool,
- light cool clothing,
- cool ambient temperature that is not too dry,
- tepid showers or baths, and
- avoid alcohol and spicy foods.

Lymphedema

Definition

Lymphedema is a chronic swelling primarily due to a failure of regional lymphatic drainage.

Prevalence

Lymphedema in cancer patients is usually caused by an obstruction or the interruption of the lymphatic system as a result of surgery, radiotherapy, or a tumor. The prevalence varies depending on the patient group and the treatment given.

For example, 30% of women who have had axillary dissection can develop lymphedema [95]. Lymphedema is more common in women than men, and there is an increase in rate with age; other risk factors include obesity and a lack of physical exercise [96].

Assessment

Although lymphedema is a chronic condition that usually affects the limbs, it can affect the trunk, head, or genital area. The skin becomes hard and thickened through fibrosis, and over time the limb becomes grossly swollen with coarsening, folding, distortion of the skin, and elephantiasis. These progressive changes are described by the International Society of Lymphology grading system (Figure 4.34) [97].

An accurate diagnosis of lymphedema is essential for appropriate therapy [98]. In most patients, the diagnosis can be readily determined from the clinical history and physical examination. Obesity, venous insufficiency, occult trauma, and repeated infection may complicate the clinical picture [99].

Grading for lymphedema	
Grade 1	Minimal or no fibrosis Edema pits on pressure Edema reduces on limb elevation
Grade 2	Substantial fibrosis Edema does not pit on pressure Edema does not reduce with limb elevation
Grade 3	Grade 2 changes plus tropic skin changes (elephantiasis)

Figure 4.34 Grading for lymphedema. (Data from the International Society of Lymphology [97])

Typical skin changes in lymphedema

Skin change	Description
Hyperkeratosis	Build-up of horny layer of skin
Lymphangiectasia	Dilated lymph vessels that appear on the skin surface like small blisters, which if damaged can leak lymph (lymphorrhea)
Papillomas	Similar to lymphangiectasia but also contain fibrous tissue, giving them a firmer consistency. They often occur in groups, producing a cobblestone-like appearance to the skin
Increased skin creases	Can become very deep in severe swelling, causing deformity of the limb
Chronic inflammation	Leads to erythema of the skin and can be similar to chronic lipodermatosclerosis, seen in venous disease
Stemmer's sign	The inability to pick up a fold of skin at the base of the second toe in lymphedema of the leg and reflects the skin and subcutaneous changes described above

Figure 4.35 Typical skin changes in lymphedema. (Data from Keeley [99])

Assessment therefore requires the exclusion of other pathologies. Although some tests are available to aid diagnosis (e.g., lymphoscintigraphy), these are seldom appropriate in patients with advanced disease.

Although size is the obvious feature of lymphedema, many patients experience pain and discomfort that can impact significantly on their quality of life [99, 100]. Patients may also experience lymphorrhea where there is leakage of lymph through the skin (Figure 4.35). The ability to perform simple tasks such as dressing may be impaired, and many patients suffer from associated emotional and psychological problems including poor body image, embarrassment, anxiety, and depression [101].

General Management

The development of lymphedema in advanced disease is distressing for patients and their carers, and can prove difficult to manage for healthcare professionals involved in their care. Patients should be given information about lymphedema, its causes, consequences, and management options with attention to skin care, emphasizing the importance of avoiding trauma [99].

Pharmacological Management

Diuretics are rarely of help in pure lymphedema. However, they may have a part to play in the management of more complex edema where fluid retention or heart failure may contribute.

Benzopyrones (e.g., coumarin, oxerutins) have been recommended for the treatment of lymphedema. Although some evidence for a beneficial effect has been reported, this has not been confirmed by a Cochrane review, which concluded that there was no evidence to support their routine use in the management of lymphedema [102].

Corticosteroids may play a part in the management of chronic edema in advanced cancer where there is metastatic lymphadenopathy [99].

Antibiotics can have a role because patients with lymphedema are at risk of developing recurrent episodes of cellulitis [99]. Antibiotics should be continued for at least 14 days or until signs of inflammation have resolved:

- amoxicillin 500 mg tds
- add flucloxacillin 500 mg qds if *Staphylococcus aureus* infection suspected, e.g., folliculitis, pus formation, or crusted dermatitis present
- if the patient is allergic to penicillin, use clindamycin 300 mg qds.

Non-pharmacological Management

The main treatment for lymphedema is based on a combination of physical treatments including [99]:

- compression,
- massage,
- exercise, and
- skin care.

There is evidence that the combination of physical treatments is effective, and in moderate-to-severe edema therapies are often phased. Care is required, however, because some physical therapies may be contraindicated in some patients (Figure 4.36) [99].

Malignant Bowel Obstruction
Definition

Malignant bowel obstruction is a mechanical obstruction of the bowel lumen and/or peristaltic failure.

Contraindications to physical therapies		
Therapy	**Contraindication**	**Reason**
Manual lymphatic drainage	Severe arterial insufficiency	Exacerbation of problem
	Uncontrolled heart failure	Damage to skin and risk of infection
	Numbness	Painful
	Acute cellulitis	
Compression garments	Arterial insufficiency	Exacerbation of problem
	Uncontrolled heart failure	Damage to skin and risk of infection
	Distorted limb	
	Ulceration	
	Lymphorrhea	
	Numbness	

Figure 4.36 **Contraindications to physical therapies**. (Data from Keeley [99])

Differentiating the location of a bowel obstruction		
Symptom	**Proximal bowel**	**Distal bowel**
Vomiting	Bilious, watery, large amounts, no to little odor	Particulate, small volumes, foul odor, may be absent
Pain	Early symptom, periumbilical, short intermittent cramps	Late symptom, localized, deep visceral pain, long intervals between cramps, often described as cramps
Abdominal distension	May be absent	Present
Anorexia	Always	May not be present

Figure 4.37 **Differentiating the location of a bowel obstruction**. (Data from Ripamonti et al. [103]. © 2008, reproduced with permission from Elsevier)

Prevalence

Bowel obstruction is a common complication in patients with end-stage cancer, particularly in those with an abdominal or pelvic primary. The reported frequency of bowel obstruction ranges from 5% to 42% in advanced ovarian cancer and from 4% to 24% in advanced colorectal cancer. The bowel obstruction may be partial or complete and at single or multiple sites; the small bowel is more commonly involved than the large bowel [103].

Assessment

The signs and symptoms of bowel obstruction vary depending on the site of the obstruction and its cause (Figure 4.37) [103]. Typical signs and symptoms include anorexia, nausea, vomiting, abdominal distension, changes in bowel sounds, and changes in bowel habits. Abdominal pain is

Causes of bowel obstruction	
Tumor mass	Single or multiple Invasion and blockage of bowel extrinsic compression
Constipation	Impacted feces
Adhesions	Postoperative Malignant Post-radiation
Volvulus	Around tumor Around adhesions Around fistula
Ileus	Infection, peritonitis Drugs
Peritonitis **Massive ascites**	Infection, bleeding

Figure 4.38 Causes of bowel obstruction. (Data from Downing [104])

a classic symptom that occurs intermittently or continuously, varies in intensity, and is described as cramping or colicky. Patients may have multiple sites of obstruction.

It is essential to determine the underlying cause of bowel obstruction (Figure 4.38) [104], because non-malignant causes such as intra-abdominal bands or adhesions resulting from prior surgery, post-radiation fibrosis, or fecal impaction secondary to ongoing morphine use will require definitive treatment.

General Management

The goal of a palliative approach to the treatment of bowel obstruction is to minimize or eliminate obstructive symptoms in order to enhance the patient's quality of life. The treatment options for malignant bowel obstruction must be carefully explored with the patient and family (Figure 4.39) [103]. This diagnosis is often an indication of disease progression, further highlighting the progressive nature of the underlying disease. It is essential that the team provide appropriate psychosocial support as treatment decisions are made [105].

Other general measures include the following:

- Frequent mouth care is essential.
- Offer ice to suck, and small amounts of food and drinks as wanted.
- Provide a low-fiber diet.

Algorithm for assessing and managing a patient with malignant bowel obstruction

Patient presenting with symptoms of bowel obstruction and a history of cancer

Clinical assessment:
- Patient acutely ill: surgical emergency. Most patient with MBO are not a surgical emergency
- History of symptoms

Radiologic assessment CT and/or MRI:
- Diagnosis and cause of obstruction
- Site: single vs multiple
  - Large vs small bowel
  - Partial (most MBO) vs complete

Patient factors:
- Age: biologic/physiologic
- Performance status
- Stage of cancer: previous treatments, any anticancer treatment options
- Malnutrition/cachexia
- Concurrent illnesses
- Ascites

Technical factors:
- Degree of invasiveness
  - Interventional radiology
  - Endoscopy
  - Open laparotomy/laparoscopy
- Anesthetic requirements
- Risk of post-procedure complications

MBO decision making:
- Identify cause for obstruction: mechanical vs functional obstruction
- Assess the realistic ability of any symptoms
- Formulate recommendations: select the intervention(s) that will provide the best results for this patient at this time
- No obligation to recommend futile therapy

Decision-making with patient and family:
- What do they understand about their disease and where they are on their diseased trajectory?
- Determine whether symptom alleviation fits the goals of care of the patient. Explainclearly the expected potential benefits of any intervention: is this something that would be worth it to them given the risk?
- Provide a commitment to contine to care for the patient regardless of the outcome of the discussion

Figure 4.39 Algorithm for assessing and managing a patient with malignant bowel obstruction. *CT* computed tomography, *MBO* malignant bowel obstruction, *MRI* magnetic resonance imaging. (Data from Ripamonti et al. [103]. © 2008, reproduced with permission from Elsevier)

Palliative pharmacotherapy of malignant bowel obstruction	
Antiemetics	
Metoclopramide	40–60 mg
Cyclizine	150 mg
Haloperidol	3–5 mg
Levomepromazine	6.25–25 mg
Analgesics	
Morphine	Titrate dose as required
Diamorphine	Titrate dose as required
Oxycodone	Titrate dose as required
Alfentanil	Titrate dose as required
Anticholinergics	
Hyoscine (scopolamine) butylbromide	60–120 mg
Hyoscine (scopolamine) hydrobromide	0.6–1.2 mg
Prokinetic agent	
Metoclopramide	40–60 mg
Somatostatin analog	
Octreotide	300–1200 µg
Corticosteroid	
Dexamethasone	8–16 µmg

Figure 4.40 Palliative pharmacotherapy of malignant bowel obstruction. Daily dose via continuous subcutaneous injection. (Data from Sykes et al. [67] and Edmonds and Wiles [106])

- If the patient is dehydrated and not dying, intravenous rehydration may be appropriate initially.
- Subcutaneous fluids may be required for the longer-term management of symptomatic dehydration or for a patient not wanting to be admitted to hospital. Hydration of 1–1.5 L/24 h may reduce nausea, but more fluid than this can result in increased bowel secretions and worsen vomiting.
- Laxatives ± rectal treatment for constipation.

Pharmacological Management

To control the pain, nausea, and vomiting of bowel obstruction, pharmacological therapy typically involves the use of analgesics, antiemetics, and anti-secretory agents [106], usually administered by CSCI because the oral route is unreliable in most patients (Figure 4.40) [67, 106]. The early introduction of pharmacological treatment can reduce symptoms, reverse

Contraindications to surgery	
Relative	Non-symptomatic extensive extra-abdominal malignant disease (eg,widespread metastases and pleural effusion)
	Poor general performance status
	Poor nutritional status (eg, marked weight loss/cachexia, marked hypoalbuminemia, and low lymphocyte count)
	Severe cachexia
	Small bowel obstruction
	Previous radiotherapy of the abdomen or pelvis
Absolute	Patient refusal
	Previous abdominal surgery that showed diffuse metastatic cancer
	Involvement of proximal stomach
	Intra-abdominal carcinomatosis demonstrated radiologically with a contrast study revealing a severe motility problem
	Diffuse palpable intra-abdominal masses (having excluded fecal masses)
	Massive ascites which rapidly recurs after drainage

Fig. 4.41 Contraindications to surgery. (Data from Sykes et al. [67])

malignant bowel obstruction, and provide better quality of life and quality of death. The choice of medications and routes of administration must be individualized for each patient.

Non-pharmacological Management
Specific non-pharmacological management approaches include the following:
- surgery, if appropriate (Figure 4.41) [67],
- self-expanding metallic stents,
- nasogastric suction, and
- gastrostomy.

Malignant Pleural Effusion
Definition
Malignant pleural effusion is an abnormal collection of fluid between the visceral and parietal pleura due to excess fluid production or decreased absorption.

Prevalence
Approximately 5–10% of cancer patients can present with pleural effusions [107, 108], and lung and breast cancer account for approximately 50–65% of all malignant effusions. Median survival following diagnosis ranges from 3 to 12 months and is dependent on the stage and type of the

underlying malignancy [108]. The morbidity and mortality of pleural effusions are directly related to cause, stage of disease at the time of presentation, and biochemical findings in the pleural fluid.

Assessment

The clinical manifestations of pleural effusion are variable and often related to the underlying disease process. The most commonly associated symptoms are progressive dyspnea, cough, and pleuritic chest pain. Most patients present with breathlessness, which is reported in 50% of patients with malignant pleural effusions [106].

Physical findings are variable and depend on the volume of the pleural effusion. Generally, there are no physical findings for effusions <300 mL. With effusions >300 mL, findings may include the following:

- dullness to percussion,
- decreased tactile fremitus,
- asymmetric chest expansion, with diminished or delayed expansion on the side of the effusion,
- diminished or inaudible breath sounds, and
- pleural friction rub.

If a pleural effusion is suspected clinically, chest radiograph is the first investigation. Malignant effusions are diagnosed by pleural fluid cytology (Figure 4.42) [109]. If this is negative, a repeat thoracocentesis and pleural biopsy will confirm malignancy in 80–90% of effusions. Determinations of pleural fluid carcinoembryonic antigen (CEA) and amylase may be helpful in selected cases; however, 10–20% of patients with malignant pleural effusions will still not have a diagnosis. In such patients, a thoracoscopy will be required for diagnosis.

General Management

Treatment options for malignant pleural effusions are determined by the symptoms and performance status of the patient, the primary tumor and its response to systemic therapy, and lung re-expansion after pleural fluid evacuation. Approximately 25% of effusions do not require therapy because they are small and stable [110].

Pleural effusion: etiology and fluid characteristics		
Cause	Exudate/Transudate	Cytology
Inflammation of pleural surface		
Infiltration by tumor	Exudate	+
Infection, infarction, irradiation	Exudate	–
Lymphatic obstruction		
Peripheral obstruction by tumor	Exudate or transudate	+/–
Central (mediastinal) obstruction	Exudate (chylous)	–
Raised pulmonary venous pressure		
Local venous obstruction by tumor	Exudate or transudate	+/–
Cardiac failure, pericardial tamponade	Transudate	–
Other edematous conditions		
Hypoproteinemia, or renal or hepatic failure	Transudate	–

Figure 4.42 Pleural effusion: etiology and fluid characteristics. (Data from Woodruff [109])

Pharmacological Management

Malignant effusions caused by lymphomas, breast cancer, small-cell lung cancer, or ovarian cancer may respond to systemic chemotherapy or hormonal therapy.

Non-pharmacological Management

Patients with symptomatic malignant pleural effusions whose underlying cancer is unlikely to respond to systemic treatment should have their pleural fluid drained. Patients with relatively large (>1,000 mL) recurrent effusions whose symptoms resolve with drainage and whose lungs can fully expand are candidates for palliation. Two general approaches to the palliative management of symptomatic pleural effusions are chest tube drainage with the installation of a sclerosing agent, and thoracoscopic drainage of the pleural effusion under local or general anesthesia with intraoperative sclerosis of the pleural space (Figure 4.43) [106].

Patients who have received extensive prior systemic therapy and those with chemotherapy-resistant tumors, such as non-small-cell lung cancer, are not likely to respond to systemic therapy. Palliative approaches to the management of malignant pleural effusions are necessary in such patients, including the palliation of cough, chest pain, and breathlessness.

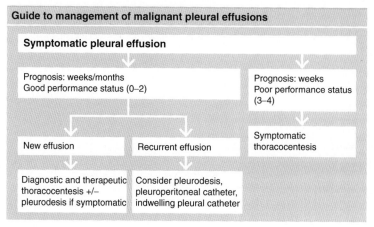

Figure 4.43 Guide to management of malignant pleural effusions. (Data from Edmonds and Wiles [106])

Malignant Wounds

Definition

Malignant wounds occur due to a malignant invasion of the epithelium and surrounding lymph and blood vessels.

Prevalence

Approximately 15% of people with metastatic cancer will develop a fungating wound [111], with 62% of these associated with breast cancer [112]. Fungating wounds tend to develop in older people, age >60 years, with advanced cancer, often within the last 6 months of life. Malignant wounds may result from direct invasion or metastatic spread. Common tumors associated with fungating wounds are breast carcinomas, sarcomas, squamous cell carcinomas, and melanomas.

Assessment

Malignant wounds may be classified into four principal classes: nodules and induration, fungating, malignant ulcers, and others. They can have a marked impact on patients [113] (Figure 4.44).

The wound should therefore be examined for the following:

• location, size, and whether it is proliferative or ulcerative,
• amount of devitalized tissue within the ulcer,

Problems arising from malignant wounds	
Psychosocial	May include depression, anxiety, poor body image, low self-esteem, and inhibited sexuality or intimacy
	Bulky dressings can affect self-image and decrease mobility
	Patients can become isolated from family and friends because of disfigurement and odor
Pain	Usually depends on the location of the wound, the depth of tissue invasion and damage, the involvement of nerves, the presence of viable tissue with exposed nerve endings, and the person's previous experience with pain and analgesia
Exudate	Can vary in amount and originates from tumor secretions and increased leakage from blood vessels
Odor	Odor occurs when tissue is deprived of oxygen and nutrients, becoming necrotic with bacterial growth
	Organisms commonly causing odor include anerobes and aerobes
	Odor can be a particular problem if the malignant ulcer is close to the bowel or the anus
	Odor can cause nausea and reduced appetite, resulting in weight loss and lethargy
Bleeding	Bleeding occurs because of abnormal microcirculation within the tumor, erosion of blood vessels by malignant cells, and decreased platelet function
Itch	Itch is different from the irritation caused by maceration and, although there may be no obvious cause, it is thought to be related to the growth of the tumor. Successful management can be difficult

Figure 4.44 Problems arising from malignant wounds. (Data from McDonald and Lesage [113])

- the condition of the surrounding skin,
- the potential for serious complications (e.g., hemorrhage), and
- complications (e.g., pain, exudate, odor, bleeding, and itch).

General Management

Explanation, education, and reassurance are required because healing, in most cases, is unlikely to be a realistic goal:

- What are the person's concerns about the wound?
- What are the factors affecting their quality of life?
- What are the person's treatment priorities?
- What are the realistic goals of treatment?

Pharmacological Management

Treatment is usually aimed at the complications of the wound (e.g., pain, infection, malodor) and may be administered orally or topically.

Local Anesthetics

For localized wound pain, topical formulations containing 2% and 4% lidocaine can be employed. These formulations have been shown to be fast acting and quite effective (lasting up to 4 h) for the management of local skin pain associated with fungating tumors.

Analgesics

A patient with malignant wounds may experience both nociceptive and neuropathic pain. Pain may be present at rest and/or during dressing changes. The appropriate drugs should be prescribed, utilizing the WHO analgesic ladder as a therapeutic tool [114]. There is some evidence that morphine administered topically to the wound can relieve pain when given as a 0.8% hydrogel mixture (10 mg morphine in 8 g of Intrasite® gel) [115].

Antibiotics

Although metronidazole can be administered orally (400 mg q8h for 7 days), a poor blood supply to the fungating wound may limit its effectiveness. Topical metronidazole can be applied using a crushed 200 mg tablet in lubricating gel, or as a commercially produced gel.

Non-pharmacological Management

Dressings

Dressings should be chosen according to the type and site of the wound, the presence of exudate or odor, comfort, and patient preference. They should be changed as often as necessary to manage odor, pain, hemorrhage, and exudate. When using dressings, do the following:

- use an appropriate size,
- carefully prepare the area around the wound, to ensure a good seal,
- do not stretch dressings or apply dressings under tension,
- protect surrounding areas of skin with a barrier if there is a risk of maceration, and
- remove dressings carefully and dispose of them safely.

Hydrogel dressings are suitable for use on lightly exuding wounds, but not for infected or heavily exuding wounds. They contain 70–90% water, and aid rehydration and autolytic debridement of dry, sloughy, or necrotic wounds. Most hydrogels need to be covered with a secondary dressing. A range of formulations is available, including gel formulations (that take up the shape of the wound) and hydrogel sheets (that have a more fixed structure) [116].

Hydrocolloid dressings aid rehydration and autolytic debridement of dry, sloughy, or necrotic wounds. They contain a variety of constituents, such as methylcellulose, pectin, gelatin, and polyisobutylene. When in contact with the wound exudate, hydrocolloids slowly absorb fluid, leading to the formation of a gel covering the wound [116].

Activated charcoal dressings can be used to absorb odor, acting as filters, binding volatile malodorous chemicals from the wound before they pass into the air. Some charcoal dressings are used as a primary contact layer (particularly if they contain other active ingredients such as alginate, hydrocolloid, or silver), and others are used as secondary dressings. As activated charcoal loses its odor-adsorbing properties once it becomes wet, frequent changes are often necessary. If the shape of the wound is awkward, it may be difficult to apply charcoal dressings because many must be applied as a sealed unit [117, 118].

Others

In selected cases the following may be considered:

- external beam radiotherapy,
- surgical debridement,
- chemotherapy,
- hormone therapy.

Fistulae

A fistula is an abnormal tract that communicates between two hollow organs. Antisecretory drugs such as anticholinergics and somatostatin analogs may be used to reduce secretions. The nursing care is similar to the principles of stoma care [119]:

- prevention of skin excoriation with barrier products,
- collection of effluent in closed stoma devices or wound management devices,
- management of odor in a closed device; the use of odor neutralizing sprays when bags are emptied or changed,

- nutrition and fluids to maintain a balance between intake and loss, which may require enteral or parenteral feeding,
- supportive care to protect the patient's sense of autonomy and ability to socialize, and
- if necessary, seek advice from a tissue viability clinical nurse specialist.

Myoclonus
Definition
Myoclonus is an intermittent, irregular, involuntary, jerking movement generally involving the limbs.

Prevalence
Myoclonus can occur as a result of immobility, pain, or other sensory stimulation. It is also a recognized side effect of opioids and is more common in patients with renal impairment [120]. Mild and infrequent myoclonus is common.

Assessment
Although myoclonus is not a life-threatening condition, it may result in serious, debilitating impairment and is frightening for both patients and their carers [121]. Although the most common time for patients to experience myoclonic jerks is while falling asleep, they are also a sign of a number of neurological disorders including multiple sclerosis, Parkinson's disease, Alzheimer's disease, subacute sclerosing panencephalitis, and Creutzfeldt–Jakob disease. In a palliative care setting, one of the most common causes is drug induced (e.g., opioids), often as a result of over-titration or renal insufficiency.

General Management
Treatment of myoclonus may not be necessary if it does not trouble the patient. If required it may be appropriate to reduce the dose of opioid, change the route of administration, or change to another opioid.

Look for reversible causes:
- correct renal failure and dehydration,
- change the opioid and decrease the analgesic dose by 20–30%,

- if renal failure is irreversible, decrease the opioid dose and the administration interval, and
- the management as above will generally resolve the problem. It is extremely unusual to require the use of benzodiazepines.

Pharmacological Management

Benzodiazepines are useful in the management of myoclonus [54]:

- Oral or subcutaneous administration of clonazepam 1 mg (500 μg in elderly people) initially at night for four nights, increased according to response over 2–4 weeks to a usual maintenance dose of 4–8 mg usually at night (which may be given in three to four divided doses if necessary).
- Oral administration of diazepam 2–15 mg/day in divided doses, increased if necessary in spastic conditions to 60 mg/day according to response.
- Midazolam 5 mg sc stat and 10 mg/24 h CSCI in moribund patients, titrating according to response.

Baclofen or dantrolene is a useful non-benzodiazepine alternative, particularly if diazepam is too sedative and anxiety is not an associated problem, or if long-term use is anticipated. The usual dosages are:

- baclofen 5 mg tds (increase to 100 mg tds), and
- dantrolene 25 mg at night (usual dose 75 mg tds).

Nausea and Vomiting
Definition

Nausea is an unpleasant sensation experienced in the back of the throat and the epigastrium that may or may not culminate in vomiting. Vomiting is the forceful expulsion of the contents of the stomach through the oral or nasal cavity. Retching is the unsuccessful attempt to vomit [122].

Prevalence

The prevalence of nausea is 20–30% in all patients with advanced cancer, and this rises to 70% in the last week of life [123]. Approximately 20% of all cancer patients develop vomiting. Nausea and vomiting are highest in advanced gynecological cancers (42%) and advanced stomach cancer (36%) [124]. Approximately 30% of patients who receive morphine feel nauseous during the first week of treatment [125].

Assessment

Although nausea, vomiting, and retching are distinct concepts, they are often used interchangeably, resulting in imprecise assessment. Furthermore, nausea or vomiting may be anticipatory, acute, delayed, or chronic, and therefore only an accurate assessment will allow for appropriate management of the patient and better symptom control (Figure 4.45) [126]:

- History: timing of symptoms, food and fluid intake, medication use, pain, bowel habit, urinary symptoms.
- Examination: hydration, infection, jaundice, neurological signs, abdominal signs, rectal examination.
- Investigations: urea and electrolytes (U&Es), corrected serum calcium level, liver function tests (LFTs), CBC and differential, urine culture, abdominal ultrasonography/radiograph, endoscopy, and CT/ magnetic resonance imaging (MRI).

General Management

Appropriate goals should be set, i.e., in patients with complete obstruction, it would be reasonable to eliminate nausea and reduce the volume and/or frequency of vomiting. General measures may include modifying the diet and the patient's environment and addressing correctable causes or exacerbating factors such as drugs, severe pain, infection, cough, and hypercalcemia. Anxiety exacerbates nausea and vomiting from any cause and may need specific treatment [127].

Pharmacological Management

First-line pharmacological treatment should be tailored according to the identified clinical syndrome and likely receptors to be targeted (Figure 4.46) [126]. Antiemetics should be used before vomiting starts (e.g., when starting opioids or chemotherapy), in adequate doses, and if necessary in combination. A non-oral route should be considered, even if only nausea is present, to ensure adequate drug bioavailability and changing to an oral preparation once the symptoms have improved. Commonly used antiemetics are listed in Figure 4.47 [54].

Other drugs used for nausea and vomiting include the following:

- Corticosteroids: dexamethasone 8–16 mg po/sc stat and daily.

Features of nausea and vomiting

Underlying cause	Examples	Mechanisms	Clinical features
Irritation or stretching of the meninges	Raised intracranial pressure caused by intracranial tumor	Unknown; may involve meningeal mechanoreceptors	Headache and nausea on lying flat, focal neurological signs, and papilledema May be confirmed by CT and MRI
Pelvic or abdominal tumor	Mesenteric metastases Metastases of liver Ureteric obstruction Retroperitoneal cancer	Stretching of mechanoreceptors	Nausea and vomiting may be caused by stretching of the mechanoreceptors. Poorly localized pain, with or without radiation, may also be present Radiology is usually required to confirm diagnosis
Bowel obstruction secondary to malignancy	Mechanical – intrinsic or extrinsic by tumor Functional – disorders of intestinal motility secondary to malignant involvement of nerves, bowel muscle, or blood supply Paraneoplastic neuropathy	Stretching of mechanoreceptors	Insidious onset and obstruction remains partial Abdominal pain is present in 90% of patients Superimposed colic in 70% Abdominal distension is less usual if the bowel is stuck down by omental metastases or in high obstruction Vomiting is an early symptom in high obstruction and may be copious. It is a later feature in large bowel obstruction Investigations are appropriate to confirm the diagnosis and constipation should be excluded
Gastric stasis	Drugs (anticholinergics, opioids) Mechanical obstruction to gastric emptying; tumor, gastritis, peptic ulcer, hepatomegaly Autonomic failure, eg, in advanced diabetes	Gastric mechanoreceptors	Fullness Epigastric pain Acid reflux Hiccups Early satiety Large-volume vomiting with little preceding nausea All symptoms are relieved by vomiting
Chemical/metabolic	Drugs – antiepileptics, opioids, antibiotics, cytotoxics, digoxin Metabolic – hypercalcemia – consider if drowsiness, confusion, thirst occurs, particularly if sudden onset Toxins, eg, tumor necrosis, bacterial toxins	Chemoreceptors in the trigger zone	The onset of symptoms may coincide with starting medication Hypercalcemia may be indicated by drowsiness (and in fact drowsiness may be the only feature in 50%) Confusion is common Polyuria and nocturia may also be present but marked if there is coincidental dehydration Blood biochemistry will confirm the diagnosis
Anxiety induced	Concern about diagnosis, treatment, symptomatology, social issues, anticipatory emesis with cytotoxics	Multiple receptors in cerebral cortex	Usually diagnosed by exclusion, and suggested by the symptoms and signs of stress
Movement related	Abdominal tumors Opioids Disease affecting vestibular system	Accentuates stretch of mechanoreceptors by tumors Vestibular sensitivity is increased Vestibular function is disturbed	Features of abdominal tumor, vestibular disease or recent commencement or increase of opioids

Figure 4.45 Features of nausea and vomiting. *CT* computed tomography, *MRI* magnetic resonance imaging. (Data from Patient UK [126])

Managing nausea and vomiting

Underlying cause Management

Irritation or stretching of the meninges	Patient with intracranial pressure, refer for radiotherapy assessment
	Trial dexamethasone (16 mg/day for 4–5 days, subsequently reducing to 4 mg/day)
	Add cyclizine 25–50 mg tds or levomepromazine on (2.5–5 mg sc or 12.5 mg po)
Pelvic or abdominal tumor	Cyclizine blocks ACh and histamine H1-receptors in vomiting center triggered by the mechanoreceptors in the abdominal and pelvic viscera Try 25–50 mg po or sc firstline, including when vomiting is aggravated by movement Add dexamethasone if vomiting persists
Partial bowel obstruction	Stop osmotic and stimulant laxatives. Titrate docusate to produce a comfortable stool without colic. Avoid high-fiber foods and advise taking food and fluids at regular intervals and in small amounts
	A prokinetic antiemetic such as metoclopramide or domperidone should be considered in patients able to pass flatus and do not have colic
	Metoclopramide 10 mg po qds or as 40–60 mg/24 hours CSCI
	Domperidone has a long plasma half-life; a starting oral dose of 20 mg bd may be increased if necessary to a 30 mg po, or 90 mg pr tds
	Prokinetic drugs should not be given with antimuscarinic drugs (eg, cyclizine, hyoscine) because they are competitively blocked by the latter. If colic develops, stop the prokinetic immediately and treat as obstruction
	Haloperidol is indicated when there is persistent vomiting or nausea in the absence of colic. Start with 2.5 mg sc. It is a specific dopamine-2-receptor antagonist that has a profoundly inhibitory effect on the CTZ
Complete bowel obstruction	First-line treatment is cyclizine, which blocks the stimulation of the vomiting center via the vagal afferents, which occurs in complete obstruction. Second line, levomepromazine
	Large-volume vomiting should be treated with an antisecretory drug
	A nasogastric tube can be inserted to drain intestinal secretions if there is gastric outflow obstruction with rapid dehydration. Intravenous/subcutaneous hydration should be considered and ranitidine can be used to reduce volume of gastric secretions
	Complete distal obstruction may require hyoscine (scopolamine) butylbromide or octreotide. Hyoscine (scopolamine) is preferred if there is colic but it is slower in reducing secretions than octreotide
	Consider referring for venting gastrostomy if there is an ongoing need for a nasogastric tube
	If vomiting persists, consider referring for stent to overcome obstruction, or consider starting corticosteroids
Gastric stasis	Prokinetics such as metoclopramide or domperidone are first-line drugs If prokinetics fail, consider adding therapies that reduce gastric secretions, such as ranitidine or octreotide

Figure 4.46 Managing nausea and vomiting (continued overleaf).

Managing nausea and vomiting

Underlying cause	Management
Chemical/ metabolic	Haloperidol is the first-line drug for opioid-induced nausea, renal failure, and hypercalcemia. Hypercalcemia should also be treated with a bisphosphonate
	A prokinetic may be useful prophylactically when initiating and titrating morphine
	If nausea develops secondary to cytotoxic therapy or radiotherapy haloperidol should be used first line, and levomepromazine second line
	Granisetron or ondansetron, specific 5HT3-receptor antagonists, block 5HT3 receptors in the gastrointestinal tract and the CNS
Anxiety induced	Ensure that all other physical causes of nausea and vomiting have been excluded before attributing the symptoms to anxiety
	Avoid diazepam, which has a long plasma half-life and may cause excessive sedation when given to palliative care patients, who may be old, debilitated, have hepatic impairment, or be on other therapy such as strong opioids
Movement related	The first-line treatment is cyclizine 25–50 mg tds. Another option is hyoscine (scopolamine) hydrobromide 300 µg po or sc or 1000 µg/ 24 hours transdermally. Cinnarizine is a further possibility
Uncertain origin	In some cases the cause of nausea or vomiting may be uncertain or where the prognosis does not warrant subjecting the patient to further invasive investigations. In such patients the use of a broad-spectrum antiemetic is appropriate such as levomepromazine, which blocks 5-HT2, histamine H1-, and ACh-receptors

Figure 4.46 Managing nausea and vomiting (continued). *ACh* acetylcholine, *bd* twice daily, *CNS* central nervous system, *CSCI* continuous subcutaneous infusion, *CTZ* chemoreceptor trigger zone, *HT* hydroxytryptamine, *po* orally, *pr* rectally, *qds* four times daily, *sc* subcutaneously, *tds* three times daily. (Data from Patient UK [126])

Commonly used antiemetics

Drug	Oral dose (rectal dose) (mg)	Stat dose/prn dose (mg)	CSCI/24 hours (mg)
Cyclizine	50 q4h–q6h	50 po/sc	50–100
Domperidone	10–20 tds/qds (30–60 tds/qds)		
Haloperidol	1.5–3 od/bd	1.5 po	2.5–5
		1.25–2.5 sc	
Levomepromazine	3–6 bd/at night	3 po	6.25–25
		2.5–6.25 sc	
Metoclopramide	10–20 tds/qds	10 po/sc	30–80
Hyoscine (scopolamine) butylbromide	20 qds	20 sc	20–100
Hyoscine (scopolamine) hydrobromide	0.15–0.3 bd/tds 1/72 hours transdermally	0.4	0.4–2.4

Figure 4.47 Commonly used antiemetics. *Bd* twice daily, *CSCI* continuous subcutaneous infusion, *od* once daily, *po* orally, *prn* as required, *qds* four times daily, *sc* subcutaneously, *tds* three times daily. (Data from Palliative Drugs [54])

- 5HT3-receptor antagonists: granisetron 1–2 mg stat and od or ondansetron 8 mg stat and bd/tds po/sc.
- Somatostatin analog: octreotide 100 µg stat, 250–500 µg/24 h CSCI, and 100 µg prn up to qds.

In the case of intractable nausea or vomiting, consider whether the assessment was adequate, the management appropriate, or the symptoms drug induced, whether autonomic failure may exist, and whether there are any unresolved psychological issues or spiritual distress.

Non-pharmacological Management

The non-pharmacological management of nausea and vomiting involves the following:

- acupuncture/acupressure,
- music therapy,
- progressive muscle relaxation, and
- guided imagery.

Pain Management
Definition

Pain is an unpleasant sensory or emotional experience associated with actual or potential tissue damage.

Prevalence

Pain remains one of the most common and most feared symptoms associated with cancer. It is prevalent in 59% of patients on active anti-cancer treatment and in 64% of patients with metastatic, advanced, or terminal disease. Furthermore, 33% of patients who have been cured of cancer also report pain [128].

Assessment

Age, gender, genetics, psychosocial context, and culture may all affect pain and analgesic efficacy. Therefore, a detailed multidimensional assessment of pain is essential and the starting point for an appropriate management plan. This should then be reviewed periodically to ensure that the plan remains relevant. A number of factors can either increase or

Factors affecting pain threshold

Aspects that lower pain tolerance	Aspects that raise pain tolerance
Discomfort	Relief of symptoms
Insomnia	Sleep
Fatigue	Rest
Anxiety	Relaxation
Fear	Explanation/support
Anger	Understanding/empathy
Boredom	Divisional activity
Sadness	Companionship/listening
Depression	Elevation of mood
Introversion	Understanding of the meaning and significance of the pain
Social abandonment	Social inclusion
Mental isolation	encouragement to express emotions

Figure 4.48 Factors affecting pain threshold. (Data from Twycross and Lack [129])

decrease the pain threshold (Figure 4.48) [129], and pain assessment should therefore extend beyond a pathophysiological evaluation to consider comorbid medical and psychosocial problems, the meaning and impact of pain on the patient and carers, and its effect on quality of life.

Types of Pain

Pain pathophysiology is one of the factors that can impact on analgesic responsiveness, and pain is broadly divided into two types – nociceptive pain and neuropathic pain.

Nociceptive pain is a normal response of the nervous system caused when a noxious stimulus (e.g., trauma, inflammation, and infection) activates Aδ-fibers and C-fibers. Nociceptive pain can be divided into somatic and visceral pain. Somatic pain is caused by the activation of nociceptors in either the cutaneous or the deep tissues. Visceral pain is caused by the activation of nociceptors resulting from infiltration, compression, extension, or stretching of the thoracic, abdominal, or pelvic viscera.

Neuropathic pain is initiated or caused by a primary lesion or dysfunction in the nervous system. The mechanisms involved in the generation of neuropathic pain are complex and include ectopic impulse generation in damaged primary afferent fibers, fiber interactions, central sensitization,

Symptoms of neuropathic pain	
	Definition
Positive	
Spontaneous pain	Painful sensations felt with no evident stimulus
Allodynia	Pain due to a stimulus that does not normally provoke pain (eg, touching, movement, cold, heat)
Hyperalgesia	An increased response to a stimulus that is normally painful (eg, cold, heat, pinprick)
Dysesthesia	An unpleasant abnormal sensation, whether spontaneous or evoked (eg, shooting sensation)
Paresthesia	An abnormal sensation, whether spontaneous or evoked (eg, tingling, buzzing, vibrating sensations)
Negative	
Hypoesthesia	Diminished sensitivity to stimulation, excluding the special senses (eg, touch, pain)
Anesthesia	A total loss of sensation (especially tactile sensitivity)
Hypoalgesia	Diminished pain in response to a normally painful stimulus
Analgesia	Absence of pain in response to stimulation that would normally be painful

Figure 4.49 Symptoms of neuropathic pain. (Data from Bennett [130])

disinhibition, and plasticity. Neuropathic pain, practically defined as pain in an area of abnormal sensation, may be associated with continuous and/or paroxysmal components, which are often described as positive or negative symptoms (Figure 4.49) that may aid diagnosis [130].

In general terms, nociceptive pains respond well to non-opioid and opioid drugs, whereas neuropathic pains may require adjuvant medication alongside conventional analgesics. A large variation may exist and the situation is further complicated when patients present with pain that has both nociceptive and neuropathic features.

Pain Assessment Tools
Examples of pain assessment tools include the Brief Pain Inventory (BPI) [124] and the Leeds Assessment of Neuropathic Signs and Symptoms (LANSS; see Appendix 2) [131]. Pain assessment questions are shown in Figure 4.50.

General Management
There are a wide variety of treatment modalities available for the management of cancer pain and their use may vary according to the primary

Pain assessment questions

	Aspect of assessment	Questions	Notes
S	Site	Where is the pain?	Consider use of body chart
O	Origin	When did the pain start?	May help with pain etiology
		How long has the pain lasted?	
		Was there a specific cause for the pain?	
C	Character	What does the pain feel like?	May help with pain pathophysiology
R	Radiation	Does the pain move anywhere?	May indicate visceral or neuropathic pains
A	Associated symptoms	Any other signs or symptoms associated with the pain?	Associated symptoms will vary according to the site and cause of the pain (eg, abdomen distension, limb weakness or numbness). May include mood symptoms such as depression
T	Time course	Does the pain follow any pattern?	Can help distinguish between background and breakthrough pain
		Does the pain remain all the time or come and go?	
		Is the pain worse at a particular time?	
E	Exacerbating/ relieving factors	Does anything make the pain worse or better?	Movement, eating (worse) Rest, analgesics (better)
S	Severity	How bad is the pain?	Consider use of pain scales

Figure 4.50 Pain assessment questions

disease, extent of disease, likely prognosis, patient preferences, and available resources. Treatment modalities should be integrated into a multi-professional plan of care with clear and realistic goals. General measures include explanation and reassurance, and lifestyle changes (e.g., pacing, aids of daily living). Management should be coordinated and consistent, and requires repeated re-assessment.

Pharmacological Management

Pharmacotherapy is the cornerstone of cancer pain treatment, with the aim of providing the greatest pain relief possible with the fewest number of adverse effects using the most convenient mode of administration. The WHO provides a simple framework for the pharmacological management of cancer pain using a stepwise approach [114] (Figure 4.51). The following are the general principles [132]:

The WHO analgesic ladder

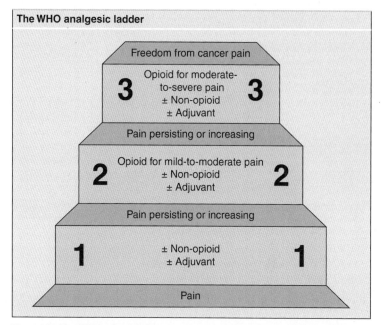

Figure 4.51 The WHO analgesic ladder. (Data from the World Health Organization [114])

- Select the appropriate analgesic drug and dose (based on the pain type and intensity).
- Administer the drug by the appropriate route (consider drug-related and patient-related factors).
- Schedule the drug by the appropriate dosing interval (consider drug-related and patient-related factors).
- Prevent background pain and relieve breakthrough pain.
- Titrate to the optimum dose that provides maximum benefit and tolerable adverse effects.
- Anticipate, prevent, and manage adverse effects.
- Consider the use adjuvant analgesics at each step.
- Review and reassess regularly.

Treatment 'by the individual' is a fundamental principle of the WHO ladder, because an individual patient's response to a particular analgesic is determined by several factors, including pain severity, previous analgesia exposure, age of the patient, extent of the cancer, and concurrent disease.

Factors increasing risk of upper gastrointestinal toxicity when NSAIDs are prescribed

- Increasing age (>65 years)
- Previous peptic ulcer disease, particularly if complicated with hemorrhage or perforation
- Comorbid medical illness
- Smoking
- Type of NSAID (eg, ketoprofen, ketorolac, and piroxicam are associated with a high risk of serious GI toxicity relative to other NSAIDs)
- Increasing NSAID dose
- Use of multiple NSAIDs
- Combined use of NSAIDs and other drugs that could increase the risk of ulceration or bleeding such as corticosteroids, anticoagulants (eg, warfarin), SSRIs, or antiplatelet agents (eg, aspirin)
- Existing renal, cardiac, or hepatic impairment

Figure 4.52 Factors increasing risk of upper gastrointestinal toxicity when NSAIDs are prescribed. *GI* gastrointestinal, *NSAID* non-steroidal anti-inflammatory drug, *SSRI* serotonin selective reuptake inhibitor. (Data from Palliative Drugs [54])

Using a simple approach in which analgesics are selected in a stepwise fashion, administering the right drug in the right dose at the right time is inexpensive and 80–90% effective [114].

Step 1: Non-opioids

The first step of the WHO analgesic ladder recommends, for mild pain (numerical rated scale [NRS] = 1–3), the use of a non-opioid with or without an adjuvant analgesic. Paracetamol (acetaminophen) is one of the most commonly used analgesics, widely available without a prescription throughout the world and, because it is well tolerated, it is widely used as the non-opioid of choice for mild cancer pain. NSAIDs are also recommended at step 1. Many preparations are available, each differing in dose, cost, drug interactions, and some specific adverse effects (Figure 4.52) [54].

Step 2: Opioids for Mild-to-Moderate Pain

The WHO ladder recommends that patients who experience moderate pain (NRS = 4–6), or fail to achieve adequate relief after a trial of a non-opioid, should be prescribed an opioid conventionally used for mild-to-moderate pain, formerly known as a weak opioid. This group of drugs includes codeine and dihydrocodeine, and at therapeutic doses there is no evidence for the superiority of one opioid over another. Non-opioids may be used with step 2 opioids, and in some countries opioid/non-opioid combinations are available and popular, largely due to convenience. Care must be taken, however, with the dose of each drug in combination formulations, because some may contain subtherapeutic doses of the opioid. In general, therefore, it is preferable to use combinations of drugs rather than combined drugs.

Step 3: Opioids for Moderate-to-Severe Pain

It is recommended that patients with severe pain (NRS = 7–10), or who fail to achieve adequate relief after appropriate administration of drug on the second step of the ladder, should be prescribed an opioid conventionally used for moderate-to-severe pain, formerly known as a strong opioid. Morphine is the most commonly prescribed step 3 opioid largely due to availability, familiarity to clinicians, established effectiveness, simplicity of administration, variety of formulations, and relatively inexpensive cost. Where possible, it should be given by mouth, with the tailored dose repeated at regular intervals so that the pain does not return. A normal-release formulation of morphine is usually preferred for dose titration and is prescribed regularly every 4 h, with extra doses permitted during the titration period as necessary. In some patients, modified-release preparations can be used during the titration process.

The starting dose for normal-release morphine is usually 5–10 mg q4h, although frail elderly patients or those with poor renal function should start with lower doses. After 24 or 48 h, the daily requirements can be reassessed and the regular dose adjusted as necessary by increasing (or decreasing) by 25–50%. This process is continued until pain relief is satisfactory.

Individualization of the dose is the key principle in opioid therapy, and patients may require regular dose adjustment. Many patients can be maintained with a modified-release preparation given once or twice daily. Patient-prescribed modified-release preparations should also be provided with a normal-release preparation to treat exacerbations of pain in-between administration of the modified-release preparation. There is no arbitrary ceiling dose of analgesia.

Although some morphine myths still persist (Figure 4.53), the drug can be used safely provided that the dose is informed by a clinical assessment.

Morphine myths

- Opioids are considered a treatment of last resort
- Opioids hasten death
- Tolerance and dependence are common
- Many patients, especially those given opioids, will exhibit 'drug-seeking' behavior
- Be very cautious in prescribing and dispensing opioids because they are associated with addiction, respiratory depression, tolerance, nausea, sedation and cognitive impairment, constipation, and regulatory concerns
- If a patient is intolerant to one opioid, they will be intolerant to all opioids

Figure 4.53 Morphine myths

If there are concerns, specialist advice should be sought rather than leaving the patient without adequate analgesia. Although morphine is generally considered the gold standard, other opioids including oxycodone, fentanyl, hydromorphone, and methadone are available [133]. Conversion tables are available [134] (Figure 4.54), but should be used with caution and only as a rough guide because a great deal of variation in dosing can exist. Whenever opioids are switched, a clinical reassessment is mandatory and the dose should be adjusted accordingly. Methadone is probably best used in a specialist setting, particularly when switching from another opioid.

Alternative Routes of Administration

Successful pharmacotherapy often depends upon the mode of drug delivery. When prescribing opioids for cancer pain the oral route is preferred, often because it is convenient and usually inexpensive. However, there are circumstances when the oral route is neither feasible nor desirable. Factors contributing to selecting an alternative administration route may be related to the patient (e.g., dysphagia, nausea, preference), pain (e.g., speed of onset, duration, and predictability), and analgesic (e.g., pharmacokinetic and pharmacodynamic profile) (Figure 4.55). Non-oral opioids may be used for titration, background, and breakthrough pain.

After opioid conversion, monitoring and dose adjustment (either up or down) according to efficacy and adverse effects are required.

Opioids can be delivered by non-oral routes such as rectal, parenteral, sublingual, buccal, nasal, and inhaled for both titration and controlled background pain [135]. When changing the route of administration and

Opioid conversions

Converting from current opioid	Converting to new opioid and/or new route of administration	Conversion*
Example		
120 mg oral morphine in 24 hours	Subcutaneous diamorphine	Divide by 3 (120/3–40 mg sc diamorphine in 24 hours)
Oral to oral route conversions		
Oral codeine	Oral morphine	Divide by 10
Oral tramadol	Oral morphine	Divide by 5
Oral morphine	Oral oxycodone	Divide by 2
Oral morphine	Oral hydromorphone	Divide by 7.5
Oral to transdermal route conversions		
Oral morphine	Transdermal fentanyl	Refer to manufacturer's information
Oral morphine	Transdermal buprenorphine	Seek specialist palliative careadvice
Oral to subcutaneous route conversions		
Oral morphine	Subcutaneous morphine	Divide by 2
Oral morphine	Subcutaneous diamorphine	Divide by 3
Oral oxycodone	Subcutaneous morphine	No change
Oral oxycodone	Subcutaneous oxycodone	Divide by 2
Oral oxycodone	Subcutaneous diamorphine	Divide by 1.5
Oral hydromorphone	Subcutaneous hydromorphone	Seek specialist palliative careadvice
Other routes rarely used in palliative medicine		
Subcutaneous or Intramuscular morphine	Intravenous morphine	No change
Intravenous morphine	Oral morphine	Multiply by 2
Oral morphine	Intramuscular morphine	Divide by 2

Figure 4.54 Opioid conversions. *To calculate the conversion divide a 24-h dose of the current opioid by the relevant figure in *column 3* to calculate initial 24-h dose of new opioid and/or new route (*column 2*). The same units must be used for both opioids or routes, e.g. mg morphine to mg oxycodone. (Reproduced with permission from the Scottish Intercollegiate Guidelines Network [134])

not the drug, the dose of the drug is usually adjusted. This is particularly important when switching between oral and parenteral routes if the opioid undergoes extensive first-pass metabolism. Assessment is important because the buccal, sublingual, and inhalational routes will not be useful in patients with severe cognitive impairment or comatose states, whereas the rectal route will not be useful in patients with diarrhea, colostomy, hemorrhoids, or anal fissures.

Indications for an alternative to oral drug administration

- Difficulty in swallowing
- Oral or pharyngeal lesions
- Persistent nausea or vomiting
- Poor alimentary absorption
- Intestinal obstruction
- Profound weakness or cachexia
- Comatose or moribund patient

Figure 4.55 Indications for an alternative to oral drug administration

Transdermal fentanyl conversion guide

Daily oral morphine (mg)	Fentanyl (μg/hour)	4-hourly oral morphine (mg)
30	25	5
60	25	10
90	25	15
120	37	20
180	50	30
240	75	40
300	75	50
360	100	60

Figure 4.56 Transdermal fentanyl conversion guide

Modified-release preparations for background pain are often preferred because they are more convenient. Transdermal systems are now widely accepted in the management of background pain provided that the pain is not unstable. Fentanyl (Figure 4.56) and buprenorphine (Figure 4.57) [136] can be administered in this way. Transdermal fentanyl is usually administered every 72 h (although a few patients require the patch to be replaced every 48 h) and transdermal buprenorphine patches are replaced every 4 (Transtec) or 7 (BuTrans) days.

Spinal opioid administration may be appropriate in the minority of patients who fail to obtain satisfactory analgesia despite careful titration of oral opioids, or who experience dose-limiting adverse effects. Epidural infusions can be delivered via either a percutaneous or an implanted epidural catheter. Intrathecal infusions using a totally implantable pump can be considered for patients with longer prognoses. Non-opioids have also been used spinally either alone or in combination with opioids in the treatment of intractable cancer pain.

Transdermal buprenorphine patch conversion guide		
Daily oral morphine (mg) *BuTrans*	**Transdermal buprenorphine (μg/hour)**	
12	5	120
24	10	240
48	20	480
Transtec		
84	35	840
126	52.5	1260
168	70	1680

Figure 4.57 Transdermal buprenorphine patch conversion guide. These conversions assume a dose ratio 100:1. (Adapted from Palliative Drugs [136])

When patients are unable to swallow or absorb oral opioids, systemic administration is an option and usually delivered as a continuous intravenous or subcutaneous infusion, the latter of which is more common. Any opioid available in an injectable formulation may be administered in this way.

Managing Adverse Effects

Opioid-related adverse effects include constipation, nausea, vomiting, pruritus, myoclonus, delirium, and drowsiness [137] (Figure 4.58). There is wide variation over time in the dose of opioid that can be tolerated, both between and within individuals. The ability to tolerate a particular dose depends on the degree of responsiveness of the pain to opioid analgesia, prior exposure to opioids, rate of titration of the dose, concomitant medication, and renal function [139].

When adverse effects become problematic the following options should be considered [131]:

- review and reassess pain,
- reduce dose of opioid,
- manage adverse effect,
- add adjuvant analgesic,
- switch opioid,
- switch route of administration,
- consider alternate treatment modalities, and
- seek advice.

Major opioid adverse effects and their management

Adverse effect	Management
Nausea and vomiting	Haloperidol 1.5–3 mg at night Metoclopramide 10 mg tds, consider non-oral route Domperidone 10 mg tds
Pruritus	Non-pharmacological treatments Opioid switch Cetirizine 10 mg od Ondansetron 4–8 mg bd
Sedation	Reduce opioid dose Review other sedating medications Opioid switch
Myoclonus	Opioid switch Diazepam 2 mg bd/tds Clonazepam 0.5–1.0 mg bd Dantrolene 25 mg on (usual dose 75 mg tds) Baclofen 5 mg tds (increase to 100 mg in divided doses)
Delirium	Opioid switch Haloperidol 3–5 mg daily (on or via CSCI) Diazepam 2–5 mg tds (use midazolam if CSCI required)
Constipation	Prophylactic treatment Stool softener and bowel stimulant (eg, Movicol® and senna) Rectal measures Opioid antagonists (methylnatrexone 8–12 mg sc alternate days)

Figure 4.58 Major opioid adverse effects and their management. *Bd* twice daily, *CSCI* continuous subcutaneous infusion, *od* once daily, *sc* subcutaneously, *tds* three times daily. (Data from Cherny et al. [138])

A careful evaluation is required to distinguish opioid adverse effects from comorbidity, dehydration, or drug interactions; moreover, the appearance of a new adverse effect in the presence of a stable opioid dose is unlikely to be caused by the opioid alone, and an alternate explanation should be sought.

Opioid Switching

Cancer patients with pain may sometimes not respond to increasing doses of opioids because they develop adverse effects before achieving an acceptable analgesia, or the analgesic response is poor, despite a rapid dose escalation [140]. Opioid switching is the term given to the clinical practice of substituting one strong opioid with another in an attempt to achieve a better balance between pain relief and side effects. Different types of opioid switching have been described and include:

Guidelines for switching opioids	
Use dose-conversion tables	• Dose-conversion tables can be used to calculate the dose of the new opioid
	• The table should relate to chronic pain management as those used in acute pain generally derive from single-dose studies
	• Large interindividual variability in response to various opioids exists amongst patients
	• Dose-conversion tables are only a guide and do not replace clinical assessment and reassessment
	• Incomplete cross-tolerance may complicate the process of switching
Dosing with new opioid	• Clinicians should be conservative in their calculations when switching between opioids
	• It is advisable to start the new opioid at doses lower than those predicted by the dose-conversion tables (eg, 30–50%)
	• Patients should be closely monitored during the switchover period, and titrate to clinical effect.
	• If pain is not well controlled, the dose can be increased
	• If the patient experiences adverse effects such as excessive somnolence, the dose may need to be titrated down

Figure 4.59 Guidelines for switching opioids. (Adapted from Cherny et al. [137])

- Switching the opioid but not the route of administration.
- Switching the route of administration of the same opioid.
- Switching both the opioid and the route of administration.

The reasons for switching include uncontrolled pain and adverse effects (either together or separately), clinical change (patient no longer able to take oral medication), and convenience.

Opioid switching should be undertaken with caution because the dose-equivalence tables that are available are a guide to switching between opioids when pain is controlled and usually describe low doses (Figure 4.59) [140]. In patients for whom pain is uncontrolled, there are adverse effects, and high doses of opioids are being given, the conversion factor between two opioids can vary widely between individuals and within the same individual, depending on which opioid is given first. In the case of methadone, the conversions have been shown to vary depending on the dose of the previous opioid. If there is any doubt, specialist help should be sought.

Tolerance, Addiction, and Physical Dependence

Tolerance to opioids is rarely seen in the clinical practice of managing cancer pain. Requirements for increasing doses of opioid can usually be

Barriers to pain control	
Healthcare professionals	Inadequate knowledge of pain management
	Poor assessment of pain
	Concern about regulation of controlled substances
	Fear of patient addiction
	Concern about side effects of analgesics
	Concern about patients becoming tolerant to analgesics
	Reluctance to report pain (concern about distracting physicians from treatment of underlying disease, fear that pain means disease is worse, concern about not being a "good" patient)
Problems related to patients	Belief that pain is inevitable
	Reluctance to take pain medications (fear of addiction or of being thought of as an addict, worries about unmanageable side effects, concern about being tolerant to pain medications)
	Physical inability to take prescribed medication
Problems related to the healthcare system	Low priority given to cancer pain treatment Restrictive regulation of controlled substances Problems of availability or accessibility of treatment

Figure 4.60 Barriers to pain control. (Adapted from the International Association for the Study of Pain [141])

explained by increases in physical activities or, more commonly, due to progressive disease.

Addiction is a psychological phenomenon consisting of three elements: loss of control, continuation despite significant adverse consequences, and the preoccupation or obsession with obtaining, using, and recovering from the effects of the drug. Addiction is not usually a problem in most patients with cancer pain but may be an issue in patients with a pre-existing addiction.

Opioids, similar to many different classes of drugs, can cause physical dependence. The body makes changes to adapt to the opioids, which if stopped suddenly can result in a withdrawal syndrome in some patients that usually manifests as a flu-like illness.

Barriers to Pain Control

Although it has been demonstrated that pain can be adequately controlled for the great majority of patients using the WHO guidelines, surveys indicate that many patients still suffer significant pain. Barriers that may interfere with adequate pain control have been broadly classified as problems related to healthcare professionals, patients, and the healthcare system (Figure 4.60) [141].

The challenge is to believe the patient, accurately assess the type and severity of pain, and choose the appropriate treatment modalities through continuity of care. To meet these challenges the following should be considered:

- improved knowledge of healthcare professionals,
- good verbal and written communication with the patient and other healthcare professionals,
- patient and carer education to reassure about pain relief and discourage acceptance of pain,
- clear planning with honest and realistic goals, and
- encouragement of patient and carer participation throughout.

Adjuvant Analgesics

Adjuvant analgesics are drugs with a primary indication other than pain but that have analgesic properties in some painful conditions [138]. They are used to enhance the analgesic efficacy of opioids, treat symptoms that exacerbate pain, and help balance the dose-related adverse effects of opioids. The term is also used to refer to other agents that should be prescribed concurrently with opioids for management of side effects (e.g., antiemetics, laxatives).

The group of adjuvant analgesics includes numerous drugs in diverse classes and can be extremely important for those patients whose pain is only partially responsive to opioids [133]. Some adjuvant analgesics are useful in several painful conditions (e.g., antidepressants), whereas others are specific for neuropathic pain (e.g., anticonvulsants), bone pain (e.g., bisphosphonates), musculoskeletal pain (e.g., muscle relaxants), or pain from bowel obstruction (e.g., anticholinergics). Adjuvant analgesics can be used at each of the three steps of the analgesic ladder. However, their use is often guided by anecdotal experience and more evidence is required to determine the most effective use of these drugs (Figure 4.61) [142].

Adjuvant Therapies
Radiotherapy

Over 50% of cancer patients receive radiotherapy and, in a third of cases, the treatment is palliative. It may be considered in a number of painful conditions, and the aim is to relieve pain quickly with the lowest possible dose and the fewest treatment fractions:

- bone metastases,
- nerve entrapment,
- fungating wound,
- dysphagia,
- pelvic tumor pain,
- chest tumor pain,
- raised intracranial pressure,
- venous obstruction,
- lymphatic obstruction,
- spinal cord compression (SCC).

Adverse effects can occur and include nausea, vomiting, diarrhea, esophagitis, alopecia, mucositis, and dry mouth. The incidence and type of adverse effects depend on the site and dose of radiation.

Adjuvant analgesics		
Type of pain	Adjuvant treatment	Dosage
Bone pain	NSAIDs	If pain is severe, or if patient has pain at rest, starting at step 3 of the WHO analgesic ladder is justified, combining a strong opioid with paracetamol (acetaminophen) or an NSAID
	Bisphosphonates	Sodium clodronate 1600 mg/day as a single dose or in two divided doses; max 3200 mg daily. Some sources recommend a 1.5 g intravenous loading dose
		Disodium clodronate 1040–2080 mg/day as a single dose or in two divided doses
		Disodium pamidronate 90 mg by slow infusion every 4 weeks (may be given every 3 weeks in breast cancer to coincide with chemotherapy)
		Zoledronic acid and ibandronic acid have also been used to treat bone pain
Bowel colic	Antispasmodic	Hyoscine (scopolamine) butylbromide 20 mg qds po Hyoscine (scopolamine) butylbromide 10–25 mg up to tds sc, iv, or im

Figure 4.61 Adjuvant analgesics (continued opposite).

Adjuvant analgesics

Type of pain	Adjuvant treatment	Dosage
Muscle spasm	Muscle relaxant	Diazepam 5 mg on (range 2–10 mg on). Using a single dose at night is recommended to reduce the impact of side effects such as drowsiness. However, some sources recommend 5 mg bd/tds po or pr
		Baclofen initially 5 mg tds, increasing by 5 mg tds at 3-day intervals as required; max 100 mg/day
Neuropathic pain	Corticosteroids	Pain caused by nerve compression may be relieved by corticosteroids, eg, dexamethasone 4–8 mg od. Corticosteroids may also be used to relieve pain caused by spinal cord compression, eg, dexamethasone 12–16 mg od
	TCAs	Amitriptyline 10–25 mg at night, titrating gradually upwards until pain controlled; maintenance 25–75 mg at night
		Imipramine, nortriptyline – 10 mg in the evening, titrating gradually upwards until pain controlled; maintenance 25–75 mg at night
	Anticonvulsants	Pregabalin initially 150 mg/day in two or three divided doses
		Increase if necessary after 3–7 days to 300 mg, then to max 600 mg daily if needed after a further 7 days
		Gabapentin: day 1 – 300 mg od, day 2 – 300 mg bd, day 3 – 300 mg tds or start at 300 mg tds on day 1. Then increase by 300 mg/day every 2–3 days to max 3600 mg/day in three divided doses
		Sodium valproate 200–500 mg in the evening, increasing to 1.5 g/day if required. Other sources recommend starting dose of 100 mg bd, increasing by 200 mg/day at 3-day intervals; usual maintenance 1–2 g/day
		Carbamazepine: use same dose as for epilepsy. Alternatively, week 1 – 100 mg in the evening, week 2 – 100 mg bd, week 3 –100 mg tds, week 4 – 200 mg bd, then 200 mg tds; maintenance 200 mg bd/qds
	NMDA receptor channel blockers	Ketamine – dosage recommendations vary. May be given po, sc, or CSCI. Suggested oral dose: 10–25 mg tds to qds increasing in 10–25 mg increments up to 50 mg qds
		Methadone – may be useful in neuropathic pain because of its possible NMDA antagonist properties

Figure 4.61 Adjuvant analgesics (continued). *Bd* twice daily, *CSCI* continuous subcutaneous infusion, *im* intramuscularly, *iv* intravenously, *NMDA* N-methyl-D-aspartate, *NSAID* non-steroidal anti-inflammatory drug, *po* orally, *pr* rectally, *qds* four times daily, *sc* subcutaneously, *tds* three times daily, *WHO* World Health Organization. (Data from MIMS [142]. Reproduced with permission from the Monthly Index of Medical Specialities)

Chemotherapy

Cytotoxic drugs cause direct damage to cells and are most useful against actively dividing cells. Cytotoxics fall into a number of classes including alkylating agents, cytotoxic antibiotics, antimetabolites, vinca alkaloids, and etoposide. Each class has its characteristic antitumor activity, sites of action, and toxic effects. Cytotoxics may be used either singly or in combination. Although not all tumors respond to chemotherapy, the relief of pain is a likely effect in those tumors that do. Adverse effects are common and include nausea, vomiting, mucositis, bone marrow suppression, bleeding, infections, and alopecia. It is important to clarify the objectives and treatment plan at the outset, and review and revise treatment based on the progress, including troublesome adverse effects.

Hormone Therapy

In some cancers, hormones can modify the pathological process and thus relieve pain. The effect is thought to be due to interactions with specific tumor receptors. Two examples include breast cancer, where approximately half of all patients benefit from hormone therapy, and prostate cancer, where a lowering of plasma male hormones can help most patients.

Surgery

There are a number of instances where surgical intervention should be considered in patients presenting with cancer-related pain:

- relief of intestinal obstruction,
- relief of urinary obstruction,
- decompression of spinal cord,
- internal fixation of pathological fracture,
- prophylactic internal fixation of bone metastases,
- cordotomy,
- pituitary ablation,
- oophorectomy,
- orchidectomy,
- resection of solitary metastases,
- resection of brain tumor,
- debridement of necrotic wound, and
- incision and drainage of abscess.

Patients may also present with pain from concurrent disorders normally requiring surgical management (e.g., appendicitis and perforated viscus). Patients considered for surgery are usually stable (unless the operation is carried out as an emergency), have limited disease, and are agreeable to this option. Surgery is usually inappropriate in patients with widespread disease and poor performance status.

Anesthetic Procedures

A number of treatment modalities may be offered via pain clinics, such as drug treatment, nerve block, nerve stimulation (e.g., acupuncture, transcutaneous nerve stimulation, and implanted stimulators) and psychological techniques. Among the nerve blocks, several can complement oral medication. They may be particularly helpful when pain is controlled at rest but not on movement, or where localized pain breaks through otherwise well-controlled pain. Agents used include local anesthetics (e.g., bupivacaine), neurolytic agents (e.g., phenol, alcohol, and glycerol), and physical agents (e.g., cryoanalgesia and radiofrequency).

Psychological therapies can be helpful for healthcare professionals to understand how each patient copes with pain, and can support and encourage the patient to develop pain-coping skills:

- individual and group counseling,
- biofeedback,
- relaxation techniques,
- self-hypnosis,
- visual imaging, and
- learning or conditioning techniques.

Support from family caregivers is also important, because they can be of assistance in helping patients identify effective coping strategies and encouraging them to use them when experiencing pain. Patients who are having particular difficulty dealing with pain may benefit from educational or psychosocial treatments designed to improve their pain-coping skills. Some psychological therapies can help reduce pain or help in coping with the effects of pain.

Physiotherapy

Physiotherapy uses physical approaches to promote, maintain, and restore physical, psychological, and social wellbeing, taking account of variations

Physiotherapy for cancer pain	
Touch therapies	Massage
	Aromatherapy
	Reflexology
Healing and energy therapies	Reiki
	Spiritual healing
	Therapeutic touch
	Hypnosis and hypnotherapy
	Acupuncture
	Homeopathy

Figure 4.62 Physiotherapy for cancer pain

in health status. Therapists adopt a patient-centered approach while working as part of the multidisciplinary team. Physiotherapy (Figure 4.62) can minimize some of the effects that the disease or its treatment has on patients, improving quality of life, regardless of their prognosis, by helping patients to achieve their maximum potential of functional ability and independence or gain relief from distressing symptoms including pain.

Complementary Therapies

Complementary therapies are often used to describe a variety of treatments employed alongside, or integrated with, orthodox medical treatment. Surveys show that over 30% of people with cancer use complementary therapies, with most in hospices and hospitals, and with up to 20% based in the voluntary sector. The touch therapies, such as aromatherapy, massage, and reflexology, are provided in over 90% of services; mind–body therapies, e.g., relaxation and visualization, in over 80%; and healing and energy work by approximately 45% of service providers [143]. A variety of complementary therapies can be helpful for cancer pain; a careful assessment should be undertaken beforehand to clarify benefits, risks, adverse effects, and interference with conventional therapies.

Breakthrough Pain

Definition

Breakthrough pain is defined as a transient exacerbation of pain that occurs either spontaneously or in relation to a specific predictable or unpredictable trigger, despite relatively stable and adequately controlled background pain [144].

Prevalence

The reported prevalence of breakthrough pain has varied from 20% to 95% [145]. Pain may be predictable or unpredictable and feels similar to background pain, although usually more severe. Patients may experience up to four episodes daily, which should be distinguished from uncontrolled background pain.

Assessment

Breakthrough pain is a heterogeneous phenomenon that is incapacitating, debilitating, and can have a significant impact on quality of life. Similar to background pain, the pathophysiology of breakthrough pain may be visceral, somatic, neuropathic, or mixed, and the etiology may be directly due to the cancer or the cancer treatment, or it may be unrelated to the cancer. Breakthrough pain is characteristically [145]:

- of rapid onset (peaks within 1–3 min),
- of moderate-to-severe intensity,
- of short duration (median 30 min, range 1–240 min),
- associated with worse psychological outcomes,
- associated with poor functional outcome,
- associated with a worse response to regular opioids, and
- associated with negative social and economic consequences.

Two breakthrough pain subtypes exist, namely incident pain and spontaneous pain (Figure 4.63).

Breakthrough pain should be distinguished from background pain, in particular uncontrolled background pain, because in most cases

Breakthrough pain subtypes	
Subtype	**Characteristics**
Incident	
Predictable	Consistent temporal relationship with predictable motor activity such as movement, micturition, breathing
Unpredictable	Inconsistent temporal relationship with motor activity such sneezing, bladder spasm
Idiopathic/ spontaneous	Not associated with a known cause, generally of longer duration than incident pain

Figure 4.63 Breakthrough pain subtypes

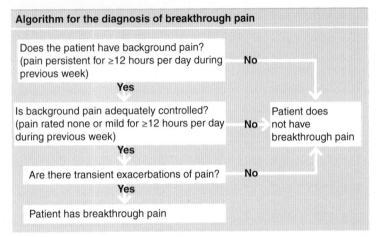

Figure 4.64 Algorithm for the diagnosis of breakthrough pain. (Data from Davies et al. [144])

Management of breakthrough pain	
Lifestyle changes	**Coping strategies**
Modification of the pathological processes	Anti-neoplastic therapies
Management of reversible causes	Incident pain precipitants
Symptomatic management of breakthrough pain	Pharmacological and non-pharmacological
Reassessment	Re-evaluation of pain and management

Figure 4.65 Management of breakthrough pain. (Data from Zeppetella [146])

background and breakthrough pain will be related (Figure 4.64) [144]. No validated tool for the clinical assessment of breakthrough pain currently exists. However, breakthrough pain is usually characterized according to its location, severity, temporal characteristics, relationship to the fixed schedule analgesic regimen, precipitating factors, predictability, pathophysiology, etiology, and palliative factors (see Appendix 2).

General Management

Successful management of breakthrough pain is best achieved by thorough assessment, good communication, reassurance about pain relief, and encouragement of patient and carer participation. Treatment should be integrated into the overall plan of care, involve pharmacological and non-pharmacological modalities, and be appropriate for the stage of disease (Figure 4.65) [146].

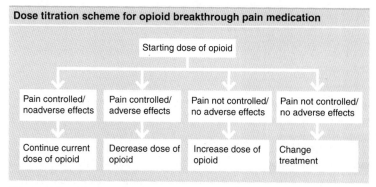

Figure 4.66 Dose titration scheme for opioid breakthrough pain medication. (Data from Davies et al. [144]. © 2009, Elsevier)

A recent expert group (Association for Palliative Medicine [APM] of Great Britain) has made recommendations about the assessment and management of breakthrough pain (Figure 4.66) [144]:

1. Patients with pain should be assessed for the presence of breakthrough pain.

2. Patients with breakthrough pain should have this pain specifically assessed.

3. The management of breakthrough pain should be individualized.

4. Consideration should be given to treatment of the underlying cause of the pain.

5. Consideration should be given to avoidance/treatment of the precipitating factors of the pain.

6. Consideration should be given to modification of the background analgesic regimen/round-the-clock medication.

7. Opioids are the rescue medication of choice in the management of breakthrough pain episodes.

8. The dose of opioid rescue medication should be determined by individual titration.

9. Non-pharmacological methods may be useful in the management of breakthrough pain episodes.

10. Non-opioid analgesics may be useful in the management of breakthrough pain episodes.

11. Interventional techniques may be useful in the management of breakthrough pain.
12. Patients with breakthrough pain should have this pain specifically reassessed.

Pharmacological Management

There is currently no 'gold standard' for the pharmacological symptomatic treatment of breakthrough pain. However, it is essential to individualize management by first considering primary therapies (e.g., radiotherapy, chemotherapy, or surgery), ensuring that round-the-clock analgesia is optimized, and providing specific analgesia for breakthrough pain. Given the heterogeneous nature of breakthrough pain, a combination of strategies may be required and the most common is the use of supplemental doses of medication known as rescue medication.

Oral opioids are the most commonly used rescue medication and normal release formulations of morphine, hydromorphone, or oxycodone are among those most frequently used. The most effective dose of rescue medication remains unknown. A fixed proportion of the round-the-clock opioid dose is usually advised, typically 10–15%. However, given that breakthrough pains may vary in etiology, intensity, and duration, it also is possible that the effective dose of rescue medication varies in each individual. It has been recommended, therefore, that the dose may require adjustment based on the balance of analgesic and adverse effects (see Figure 4.64) [144].

An orally administered opioid rescue dose often has an onset of meaningful analgesia up to an hour after administration and a duration that may last 4 h or more. Hence, it may not be ideal for breakthrough pain that peaks rapidly and persists for less than 1 h. Patients may therefore obtain very little or delayed relief, even when rescue medication is used prophylactically, or adverse effects may become problematic due to the effects of the medication that persist long after the pain has resolved. The mismatch between pharmacokinetics and the time course of the pain has driven the development of transmucosal opioid formulations that may have a more rapid onset of effect.

More recently, transmucosal opioid formulations specifically developed for the management of breakthrough pain have been introduced (Figure 4.67). Transmucosal formulations comprise a variety of delivery systems that

Transmucosal opioid formulations

Preparation (brand name)	Formulation	Manufacturer	Available strengths (μg)
Oral transmucosal fentanyl citrate (OTFC, Actiq)	Buccal lozenge on a stick	Cephalon	200, 400, 600, 800, 1200, 1600
Fentanyl buccal tablet (Fbt, effentora, Fentora)	Effervescent buccal tablet	Cephalon	100, 200, 400, 600, 800
Fentanyl orally disintegrating tablet (ODT, Abstral)	Sublingual tablet	Prostrakan	100, 200, 300, 400, 600, 800
Intranasal fentanyl spray (INFS, Instanyl)	Nasal spray	Nycomed	50, 100, 200 μg/dose
Fentanyl pectin nasal spray (FPNS, PecFent)	Nasal spray	Archimedes	100, 400 μg/spray
Fentanyl buccal soluble film (FBSF, Onsolis)	Buccal soluble film	MEDA Pharmaceuticals	200, 400, 600, 800, 1200

Figure 4.67 Transmucosal opioid formulations

present the drug to the oral or nasal mucosa, and offer the potential for a more rapid onset of action [147]. The evidence suggests that the successful dose of these formulations does not correspond to the around-the-clock dose. Accordingly, it is recommended that treatment with these formulations always start with a low dose, which should then be titrated to identify the effective dose. As titration schedules vary from one product to another it is important to check the individual product's data sheet [148]. Patients switching from one transmucosal formulation to another may require re-titration.

Non-pharmacological Management

Non-pharmacological approaches should be considered in the management of breakthrough pain, and patients often volunteer that such treatments are helpful. Some require healthcare professionals, such as an occupational therapist, physiotherapist, clinical psychologist, or chronic pain nurse. Patients have reported a number of helpful therapies, including massage, application of heat or cold, distraction therapies, and relaxation techniques. Related cognitive–behavioral strategies might also be considered, and other physical medicine or complementary strategies, such as therapeutic exercise, transcutaneous electrical nerve stimulation, and acupuncture, can also play a role. These non-pharmacological strategies can be tried either before, or alongside, pharmacological therapy [149].

Rectal Tenesmus
Definition
Rectal tenesmus is a feeling of incomplete defecation that is frequently painful and may be accompanied by involuntary straining and other gastrointestinal symptoms.

Prevalence
The prevalence of tenesmus has not been accurately documented but is most commonly encountered in patients with carcinoma of the rectum or other pelvic organs.

Assessment
Tenesmus may be related to cancer or cancer treatment, or be independent of them (Figure 4.68) [150], and during the course of the assessment a number of questions may be helpful in differentiating etiologies:

- When did the problem start?
- Is there a constant urge to empty the bowels, or is the feeling intermittent?
- How much tends to be passed?
- Is there abdominal pain? If so, where?
- Is there a great urge to strain?
- Is there diarrhea or vomiting?
- Is any blood passed?
- Have you eaten anything unusual or been somewhere where there is a risk that the food may produce gastroenteritis?
- Have any family or close friends had similar problems?
- Are there any medical problems?

If the cause of tenesmus is not apparent routine blood tests may help exclude an underlying inflammatory condition. In some cases, sigmoidoscopy or even colonoscopy may be required, although a plain abdominal radiograph can be of value.

Causes of tenesmus	
Symptom	**Cause**
Pain alone	Anal fissure Anal herpes Ulcerative proctitis Proctalgia fugax
Bleeding alone	Internal hemorrhoids Colorectal polyps Colorectal carcinoma Anal carcinoma
Lump alone	Skin tags Perianal warts Anal carcinoma
Pain and lump	Perianal hematoma Strangulated internal hemorrhoids Perianal or ischiorectal abscess Pilonidal sinus
Pain and bleeding	Anal fissure Proctitis
Lump and bleeding	Second-degree hemorrhoids Anal carcinoma
Pain, lump and bleeding	Second, third, and fourth degree hemorrhoids Ulcerated perianal hematoma

Figure 4.68 Causes of tenesmus. (Data from Daniel [150])

General Management

Management will depend on the cause. Consideration should also be given to the anxiety and fear associated with defecation, which, even if successful, can cause a worsening of the pain.

Pharmacological Management

Tenesmus has both nociceptive and neuropathic elements. Non-opioids and opioids are often trialed first (in some cases an opioid switch may be required) [151]; however, it is not uncommon for the patient to require additional management strategies including [54]:

- adjuvant analgesics as for neuropathic pain (e.g., amitriptyline, pregabalin),

- corticosteroids (e.g., dexamethasone 8–12 mg/day), and
- calcium-channel blockers (modified-release nifedipine 10–20 mg bd).

Non-pharmacological Management

Non-pharmacological management of tenesmus involves:

- radiotherapy,
- nerve block,
- endoscopic laser therapy, and
- a self-expandable metal stent.

Stomatitis
Definition

Stomatitis is a diffuse inflammatory, erosive, and ulcerative condition that affects the mucous membranes of the mouth. The term 'mucositis' is often used synonymously with stomatitis, but refers to the inflammatory reaction caused by chemotherapy or local radiotherapy, which can occur throughout the gastrointestinal tract.

Prevalence

Stomatitis has been reported in up to 40% of all patients receiving chemotherapy and up to 80% of patients having local radiotherapy for head and neck tumors [152]. Seventy-five percent of patients with stomatitis complain of oral pain [153].

Assessment

A number of grading tools are available for the assessment of patients with stomatitis, one of which is the WHO grading for mucositis/stomatitis (Figure 4.69) [154, 155].

The causes of ulceration of the oral mucosa include trauma, recurrent aphthous ulcers, infection, cancer, and nutritional deficiencies. It is important to determine the cause so that, if appropriate, specific as well as symptomatic treatment is given. Mucositis tends to heal 2–3 weeks after the course of chemotherapy or radiotherapy treatment has finished. As patients are prone to develop other mouth problems such as infection and dry mouth, specific treatments may be required.

WHO grading of stomatitis	
Grade	Symptom
0	None
I	Painful ulcers, erythema, or mild soreness
II	Painful ulcers, edema, or ulcers but able to eat
III	Painful ulcers, edema, or ulcers, unable to eat
IV	Requires parenteral or enteral support

Figure 4.69 WHO grading of stomatitis. (Reproduced with permission from the World Health Organization [145])

General Management

Meticulous oral care can reduce the severity of stomatitis [79]. The primary preventive measures include good nutritional intake, good oral hygiene practices, and early detection of any oral lesions by either the patient or a healthcare professional. The following measures may be recommended to treat stomatitis:

- Rinse the mouth after meals and before bedtime to ensure that it is clean and free of debris.
- Use a soft-bristled toothbrush or soft foam tooth-cleaning device to clean the mouth and teeth.
- Maintain good nutritional intake.
- Drink adequate amounts of fluids.
- Avoid tobacco and alcohol.
- Avoid spicy, acidic, or very hot foods.
- Dentures should be removed at night and carefully cleaned with an antiseptic solution.

Other prophylactic interventions that have been shown to either prevent or reduce the severity of mucositis include allopurinol, aloe vera, amifostine, cryotherapy, intravenous glutamine, honey, keratinocyte growth factor, laser, and polymixin/tobramycin/amphotericin antibiotic pastille/paste [156].

Pharmacological Management

If the mouth sores are painful enough to prohibit eating and drinking, analgesics (either topically or systemically) may be required. Topical non-opioid analgesics have a relatively short duration of action. Benzydamine (an NSAID with antimicrobial and mild local anesthetic effects) is available as an oral rinse or spray to ease the discomfort associated with various causes of sore mouth, including chemotherapy and radiation therapy. Choline salicylate dental gel provides similar relief. Other options include diclofenac dispersible tablets, 50 mg tds, which should be swished around the mouth for 5 min before swallowing. Flurbiprofen lozenges (8.75 mg q3h–q6h prn) are suitable for oral and pharyngeal pain. The maximum recommended dose is five lozenges/24 h.

Topical local anesthetics may also be used such as lidocaine ointment 5% (has a water-miscible base), applied as needed and benzocaine suspension 150 mg/5 mL (available as a special order; sip 5–10 mL slowly so that it coats the mouth and pharynx).

Topical opioids have a topical analgesic effect on inflamed tissue and can be used as a mouthwash [157]. Some recommend that the mouthwash be subsequently swallowed in order to combine a systemic analgesic effect with the topical one. Morphine sulfate solutions, extemporaneous (0.2%, i.e., 2 mg in 1 mL water) or an alcohol-free proprietary preparation, 10 mg q3h–q4h, hold in the mouth for 2 min and then spit out or swallow; some patients need higher doses, occasionally 30 mg q3h–q4h.

Systemic non-opioid and opioid analgesics may be appropriate for severe mucositis inadequately relieved by topical measures. A parenteral opioid should be administered, e.g., morphine [158]. Chemotherapy patients often have a permanent intravenous access (e.g., Hickman line), and this can be used for patient-controlled analgesia. In other patients and in palliative care generally, CSCI is likely to be more convenient.

A step-wise approach is often advised [54]:

- Topical non-opioid analgesic.
- Topical local anesthetic ± topical non-opioid analgesic.
- Topical morphine ± systemic morphine.
- Concurrent use of 'burst' ketamine.
- Concurrent use of thalidomide.

Non-pharmacological Management

A number of complementary therapies have been used for stomatitis. Some preliminary studies have shown that the amino acid glutamine can be effective in shortening the duration of stomatitis, as well as topical vitamin E. Other small studies suggest that using ice chips or a chamo-mile mouthwash will decrease the severity of symptoms.

Sweating
Definition
Sweating is a mechanism that the body uses to maintain normal physio-logical temperature.

Prevalence
Excessive sweating occurs in an estimated 16–28% of patients with cancer [159] and can present as either focal (confined to the forehead, feet, palms, or armpits) or generalized (sweating that occurs all over the body, not just limited to the focal areas). Sweating problems can occur throughout the day, but generally worsen at night, contributing to sleep disturbances.

Assessment
Excessive sweating results in feelings of self-consciousness and may con-tribute to or cause health problems, such as dehydration or salt imbalance [160]. Sweat on the skin's surface also acts as a breeding ground for bac-teria, especially between skin folds, which may develop into skin infec-tions. There are multiple causes of excessive sweating (Figure 4.70) [94].

General Management
General management of sweating involves the following [161]:
- treat any underlying cause,
- reduce room temperature, remove excess bedding, increase ventilation, and use a fan,
- wear loose cotton clothing, cool with tepid sponging,
- maintain fluid intake to avoid dehydration, and
- review medication and prescribe an alternative if possible.

Pharmacological Management
For the pharmacological management of sweating with pyrexia:
- paracetamol (acetaminophen) 1 g qds,
- NSAIDs.

Causes of excessive sweating	
Localized	**Generalized**
Essential (primary)	Systemic diseases
Neurogenic	Pheochromocytoma
Peripheral neuropathy	Thyrotoxicosis
Spinal cord disease	Hypopituitarism
Cerebrovascular accident	Diabetes mellitus
Intrathoracic neoplasm or mass	Acromegaly
Unilateral circumscribed	Hypoglycemia
Cold induced	Carcinoid syndrome
Associated with cutaneous lesions	Menopause
Gustatory	Tuberculosis
	Lymphoma
	Endocarditis
	Angina
	Malignancy
	Nocturnal
	Episodic
	Medication induced

Figure 4.70 Causes of excessive sweating. (Data from Pittelkow and Loprinzi [94])

For the pharmacological management of sweating without pyrexia (associated with tumor):

- NSAIDs (e.g., diclofenac 50 mg tds),
- dexamethasone 1–2 mg daily,
- antimuscarinics (e.g., amitriptyline 10–50 mg at night, levomepromazine 3–6 mg at night),
- gabapentin 100 mg tds,
- SSRIs (e.g., fluoxetine 20 mg od),
- cimetidine 400–800 mg od/bd.

In cases of sweating with hormone insufficiency advice should be sought from an oncologist about hormone replacement therapy.

Other

For primary localized sweating, an endoscopic thoracic sympathectomy or the administration of botulinum toxin injections into the affected skin regions is a potential treatment option [94].

Taste Disturbances

Definitions

Patients may be affected by different taste disturbances:

- ageusia: an absence of taste
- hypoeusia: a reduction in taste
- dysgeusia: a distortion of taste.

Prevalence

The prevalence of taste disturbances ranges from 25% to 50% [72].

Assessment

A number of potential causes for taste changes require consideration (Figure 4.71) [69]. Assessment includes questions about local issues such as salivation, swallowing, chewing, oral pain, oral hygiene, and stomach problems, and systemic diseases such as diabetes mellitus, hypothyroidism, or cancer. Clinical examination includes an inspection of the tongue and the oral cavity.

The duration of the symptoms of taste disturbances depends on the cause. If the alteration in the sense of taste is due to gum disease, dental plaque, a temporary medication, or a short-term condition such as a cold,

Taste disturbance in patients with cancer	
Cancer related	Local tumor infiltration
	Paraneoplastic syndrome
Cancer treatment related	Local surgery
	Local radiotherapy
	Systemic chemotherapy (eg, carboplatin)
	Topical drug treatments (eg, benzocaine)
	Systemic drug treatments (eg, amitriptyline)
Other oral problems	Dry mouth
	Poor oral hygiene
	Oral infection
Miscellaneous	Malnutrition
	Zinc deficiency
	Diabetes mellitus
	Renal disease
	Neurological disease

Figure 4.71 Taste disturbance in patients with cancer. (Data from Davies [69])

the taste disturbances should disappear once the cause is removed. After radiotherapy, taste changes can start within 2 days and remain altered for weeks or months after completion of therapy, although some patients have a permanent alteration [162].

General Management

Due to the variety of causes of altered taste, there are many possible treatments, usually requiring a multiprofessional approach. If possible, the underlying cause of the taste disturbance should be addressed (e.g., reviewing the medication). Where this is not possible, symptomatic management is provided.

Pharmacological Management

A number of different approaches are available for the pharmacological management of taste disturbances [7, 54].

Artificial Saliva

Artificial saliva mimics the characteristics of natural saliva by lubricating and protecting the mouth, but does not provide any digestive or enzymatic benefits:

- AS Saliva Orthana spray can be given two to three times on to oral and pharyngeal mucosa, when required.
- Biotène Oral Balance should be applied to the gums and tongue as required.
- Glandosane aerosol spray can be sprayed on to the oral and pharyngeal mucosa, when required.

Pilocarpine

Pilocarpine is a cholinergic drug that has the same effects as the neurotransmitter acetylcholine (ACh). The increase in saliva flow is effective in improving the movement of food to the taste buds. The recommended dose of pilocarpine is 5 mg tds. Alternatively, bethanecol 10–25 mg tds can be used.

Zinc Supplements

Zinc supplements are generally used when there is good evidence of deficiency (hypoproteinemia spuriously lowers plasma zinc concentration) or in zinc-losing conditions. Zinc deficiency can occur as a result of inadequate diet or malabsorption. Excessive loss of zinc can occur in trauma, burns, and protein-losing conditions. A zinc supplement is given until clinical improvement occurs, but it may need to be continued in cases of severe malabsorption, metabolic disease, or zinc-losing states. An excess amount of zinc in the body can have negative effects on the immune system, and physicians must exercise caution when administering zinc to immunocompromised cancer patients. The recommended dose of zinc sulfate monohydrate is 125 mg (45 mg zinc), or one tablet in water once to three times daily after food.

Corticosteroids

Oral corticosteroids have been reported to be effective in patients with advanced cancer, although the mechanism of action is unknown. The recommended dose of dexamethasone is 2–4 mg/day.

α-Lipoic Acid

α-Lipoic acid (ALA) is an antioxidant that is made naturally by human cells. It can be administered in capsules or found in foods such as red meat, organ meats, and yeast. Similar to other antioxidants, it functions by ridding the body of harmful free radicals that can cause damage to tissues and organs. ALA has proven to be an effective treatment for burning mouth syndrome, spurring studies into its potential to treat taste disturbances.

Non-pharmacological Management

Dietary interventions:

- eat food that tastes good,
- avoid food that tastes bad,
- enhance the flavor of the food (use of sugar, salt, and other flavorings), and
- focus on smell, presentation, consistency, and temperature of the food.

Urinary Symptoms
Definition

Urinary problems include the unsatisfactory voiding of urinary from the bladder.

Prevalence

Urinary problems are increasingly prevalent as disease progresses. Up to 50% of patients can develop urinary problems during the last 48 h of life [163].

Assessment

Urinary problems can be dehumanizing and deeply degrading. The patient's underlying disease, pain, and functional and cognitive status will be the starting point for the clinical assessment. An accurate assessment of the patient's urinary symptoms, together with an understanding of the underlying disease and its complications, will prevent unnecessary interventions and reduce any potential suffering [164].

Continence difficulties may be:

- caused by an underlying condition
- triggered by medication
- associated with reduced mobility or cognitive decline
- present before the onset of the disease.

Any component of the urinary pathway can be affected and result in problems for the patient (Figure 4.72) [165].

General Management

Adequate hydration may reduce bladder symptoms associated with dehydration, urinary tract infection, or post-radiotherapy irritation. Fluid advice should be individualized and symptoms such as pain or nausea might need to be relieved before hydration can be addressed. Bladder symptoms should be considered in clinical decisions concerning the maintenance or withdrawal of hydration.

Ensuring that each patient has a regular toilet or pad regimen will help to promote comfort and dignity. A commode near the bed or the use of a bedpan or urinal can mean that a patient can remain continent until very close to the end of life. If the patient has a history of continence difficulties before the terminal illness, management may need to be reconsidered. For example, intermittent catheterization may need to be replaced with an indwelling catheter.

Common urinary problems in palliative care

Problem	Cause
Retention	Obstruction
	Enlarged prostate
	Impacted feces in rectum
	Generalized weakness
	Depression
	Lack of awareness/delirium
	Drugs
	Tricyclic antidepressants
	Morphine
	Spinal cord compression
Incontinence	
Total	Local tumor involvement
	Overflow due to urethral or catheter obstruction Confusion leading to inappropriate voiding
Stress	Weak pelvic floor, hypotonic bladder
Neurological	Hypotonic (neuropathic) bladder due to sacral plexus or spinal cord compression below T1
Other causes	Fistulae (vesicovaginal/vesicoenteric)
	Infection
	Diabetes
	Fecal impaction
Pain	Renal colic
	Obstructive bladder
	Irritative bladder pain
Discolored urine	Blood
	Drugs
	Danthron
	Senna
	Rifampicin
	Chemotherapy
	Doxorubicin
	Mitoxantrone
	Food dyes
	Beetroot
	Rhubarb
	Bile

Figure 4.72 Common urinary problems in palliative care (continued overleaf).

Common urinary problems in palliative care

Problem	Cause
Increased urine output	Drugs Diuretics Endocrine Diabetes mellitus Hypercalcemia Chronic renal failure Diabetes insipidus Anxiety and excessive drinking
Decreased urine output	Dehydration Bilateral ureteric obstruction Urethral obstruction Catheter blocked endocrine (syndrome of inappropriate antidiuretic hormonesecretion)
Frequency of urine	Causes of increased urine output Infection Unstable bladder Anxiety Obstruction with overflow Small capacity bladder due to tumor/post-radiotherapy
Decreased frequency	Causes of decreased urine output Antimuscarinic drugs Hyoscine (scopolamine) Tricyclic antidepressants Neurological problems
Catheter-related problems	Blocked catheter Bypassing of urine Infection Urethritis encrustation
Bladder spasms	Consider retention Clot retention Balloon in urethra

Figure 4.72 Common urinary problems in palliative care (continued). (Data from Swann and Edmonds [165])

Skin care is an important part of continence management in frail and immobile individuals. Barrier creams, repositioning, and constant re-evaluation are the cornerstone to preventing pressure ulcers and further discomfort. Reversible causes should be sought and treated.

Pharmacological management of selected urinary problems	
Bladder pain	**Analgesia according to the WHO analgesic ladder**
Nocturnal urinary frequency or incontinenceurge	Imipramine 10–50 mg
Stress incontinence in postmenopausal women	Dienestrol cream prn
Bladder spasms and urgency	Oxybutynin 5 mg tds
Renal colic	Diclofenac 50 mg tds Hyoscine butylbromide 20 mg tds
Intractable nocturnal incontinence	Desmopressin 100–200 µg in the evening

Figure 4.73 Pharmacological management of selected urinary problems. *Prn* as required, *tds* three times daily, *WHO* World Health Organization. (Data from Swann and Edmonds [165])

Pharmacological Management

Pharmacological management is based on the assessment and diagnosis of the urinary problem (Figure 4.73) [165]. Drugs used for urinary frequency and bladder spasms include the following [7, 54]:

- antimuscarinics are the drugs of choice, even though treatment may be limited by other antimuscarinic effects:
  - oxybutynin 2.5–5 mg bd/qds also has a topical anesthetic effect on the bladder mucosa,
  - tolterodine 2 mg bd is as effective as oxybutynin 5 mg tds, but has fewer antimuscarinic effects,
  - amitriptyline 25–50 mg at night, and
  - propantheline 15–30 mg bd/tds.
- sympathomimetics, e.g., terbutaline 5 mg tds,
- musculotropic drugs, e.g., flavoxate 200–400 mg tds,
- NSAIDs, e.g., naproxen 250–500 mg bd, and
- vasopressin analogs (e.g., desmopressin) are of value in refractory nocturia; hyponatremia is a possible complication.

Non-pharmacological Management

Indwelling catheters are a suitable option in the management of urinary incontinence, because they improve skin care where incontinence could or has caused a problem or to reduce movement and suffering. The choice of catheter will be based on the estimated time that it will be in place and any known allergies that the patient has. Catheter management at the end of life requires attention to comfort, infection prevention, and dignity. There is some evidence that silicone catheters may reduce inflammation and that basic hand hygiene, soap and water cleansing of the urethral meatus, and vigorous maintenance of a closed system reduce the risk of infection [164].

Weakness and Fatigue

Definition

Weakness and fatigue are defined as a persistent, subjective feeling of tiredness, weakness, or lack of physical or mental energy.

Prevalence

Weakness and fatigue are common and affect 70–100% of patients receiving cancer treatment [166]. They are common in the last days of life and part of a normal dying process.

Assessment

Weakness and fatigue are not related to level of activity and not alleviated by rest or sleep. They affect physical function, cognitive ability, and emotional and spiritual wellbeing. There are multiple contributory causes (Figure 4.74) [167], but, as the exact etiology is poorly understood, a com-

Associated symptoms with weakness and fatigue
• Pain
• Anxiety, depression
• Sleep disturbance
• Anemia
• Poor nutrition or absorption
• Fluid/electrolyte imbalance: check sodium, potassium, calcium, magnesium
• De-conditioning due to reduced activity level/fitness or muscle wasting
Comorbidities:
• Chronic infection
• Cardiac or respiratory disease
• Renal or hepatic impairment
• Hypothyroidism, adrenal insufficiency, hypogonadism

Figure 4.74 Associated symptoms with weakness and fatigue. (Reproduced with permission from NHS Scotland [167])

bination of management approaches, tailored to the individual patient, is needed; patients should be screened for fatigue and its impact including:

- symptom pattern, duration; associated or alleviating factors
- interference with function and quality of life
- severity: mild, moderate, or severe or rated on a 0–10 scale.

The disease status and current treatment also require assessment in order to exclude cancer recurrence or progression. Predisposing medication (e.g., hormones, β blockers, sedative drugs, corticosteroids, opioids) should also be reviewed.

General Management

An activity diary may help identify precipitants/timing of symptoms. If a reversible cause is identified this should be managed. In most instances there will be several causes, many of which will be irreversible. The reality of the symptoms and their impact on the patient and carers should be acknowledged and their understanding of the causes explored. Explanation and appropriate reassurance are important and coping strategies should be discussed.

Pharmacological Management

If a specific cause is identified during the assessment (e.g., anemia, anorexia, insomnia) this should be treated and the patient's response assessed. In patients with anorexia/cachexia-related fatigue, corticosteroids or progestogens may be helpful (see Anorexia).

Psychostimulants are occasionally used in a palliative care setting, although the evidence to support their use is of low level, and their use by non-specialists is not advised:

- Methylphenidate: start at 5 mg bd and increase over a 1-week period to 15 mg bd. If it is ineffective at that dose there is no point in continuing it.
- Modafinil: 200 mg/day, either in two divided doses in the morning and at noon or as a single dose in the morning, with the dose adjusted according to response to 200–400 mg/day in two divided doses, or as a single dose.

Non-pharmacological Management

Physical activity [168]:

- Graded exercise, both aerobic and strength training: consider physiotherapy referral.
- Energy conservation: set priorities, pace, schedule activities at times of peak energy, eliminate non-essential activities, short daytime naps if sleep at night is not affected, attend to one activity at a time, and conserve energy for valued activities.
- Psychosocial interventions: stress management, relaxation therapy, sleep hygiene.

References

1. Potter J, Hami F, Bryan T, Quigley C. Symptoms in 400 patients referred to palliative care services: prevalence and patterns. Palliat Med. 2003;17:310–4.
2. Chang VT. Tools for pain and symptom assessment in palliative care. In: Bruera E, Higginson IJ, Ripamonti C, von Gunten C, editors. Textbook of palliative medicine. London: Hodder Arnold; 2006. p. 333–48.
3. Dunn A, Carter J, Carter H. Anemia at the end of life: prevalence, significance and causes in patients receiving palliative care. J Pain Symptom Manage. 2003;26:1132–329.
4. Turner AR. Clinical management of anaemia, cytopenias, and thrombosis in palliative care. In: Hanks G, Cherny N, Kaasa S, et al., editors. Oxford textbook of palliative medicine. 4th ed. Oxford: Oxford University Press; 2010. p. 928–33.
5. Hirst B. Management of anemia in palliative care. MIMS oncology & palliative care. 2009. Available at: www.healthcarerepublic.com/News/EmailThisArticle/915238/Management-anaemia-palliative-care. Last accessed 27 Nov 2011.
6. Cook JD. Diagnosis and management of iron-deficiency anaemia. Best Pract Res Clin Haematol. 2005;18:319–32.
7. British National Formulary. BNF 61. London: BMJ Group and Pharmaceutical Press; 2011. Available at: www.bnf.org. Last accessed 27 Nov 2011.
8. Bohlius J, Wilson J, Seidenfeld WJ, et al. Erythropoietin or darbopoietin for patients with cancer. Cochrane Database Syst Rev. 2006;(3):CD003407.
9. Gleeson C, Spencer D. Blood transfusion and its benefits in palliative care. Palliat Med. 1995;9:307–13.
10. Nelson KA. Modern management of the cancer anorexia–cachexia syndrome. Curr Pain Headache Rep. 2001;5:250–6.
11. MacDonald N. Anorexia–cachexia syndrome. Eur J Palliat Care. 2005;12:8–14.
12. Fearon KCH, Baracos V, Watanabe S. Classification, clinical assessment and treatment of the anorexia–cachexia syndrome. In: Hanks G, Cherny N, Kaasa S, et al., editors. Oxford textbook of palliative medicine. 4th ed. Oxford: Oxford University Press; 2010. p. 908–15.
13. NHS Scotland. Palliative care guidelines – symptom control – anorexia. 2009. Available at: www.palliativecareguidelines.scot.nhs.uk/documents/Anorexia.pdf. Last accessed 27 Nov 2011.
14. Loprinzi CL, Michalak JC, Schaid DJ, et al. Phase III evaluation of four doses of megestrol acetate as therapy for patients with cancer anorexia and/or cachexia. J Clin Oncol. 1993;11:762–7.
15. American Psychiatric Association. Diagnostic and statistical manual of mental disorders. 4th ed. Washington, D.C.: APA; 2000.
16. Stoklosa J, Patterson K, Rosielle D, Arnold R. Anxiety in palliative care – causes and diagnosis. J Palliat Med. 2011;14:1173–4.
17. Roth AJ, Massie MJ. Anxiety and its management in advanced cancer. Curr Opin Support Palliat Care. 2007;1:50–6.

18. Zigmond AS, Snaith RP. The hospital anxiety and depression scale. Acta Psychiatr Scand. 1983;67:361–70.

19. Jacobsen PB, Donovan KA, Trask PC, et al. Screening for psychological distress in ambulatory cancer patients. Cancer. 2005;103:1494–502.

20. Breitbart W, Chochinov HM, Passik SD. Psychiatric symptoms in palliative medicine. In: Hanks G, Cherny N, Kaasa S, et al., editors. Oxford textbook of palliative medicine. 4th ed. Oxford: Oxford University Press; 2010. p. 1453–82.

21. Anderson T, Watson M, Davidson R. The use of cognitive behavioural therapy techniques for anxiety and depression in hospice patients: a feasibility study. Palliat Med. 2008;22:814–21.

22. Runyon BA. Care of patients with ascites. N Engl J Med. 1994;330:337–42.

23. Ayuntunde AA, Parsons SL. Pattern and prognostic factors in patients with malignant ascites: a retrospective study. Ann Oncol. 2007;18:945–9.

24. Becker G, Galandi D, Blum HE. Malignant ascites: systematic review and guideline for treatment. Eur J Cancer. 2006;42:589–97.

25. Chan KS, Tse MW, Sham MMK, Thorsen AB. Palliative medicine in malignant respiratory disease. In: Hanks G, Cherny N, Kaasa S, editors. Oxford textbook of palliative medicine. 4th ed. Oxford: Oxford University Press; 2010. p. 1107–44.

26. Dorman S, Byrne A, Edwards A. Which measurement scales should we use to measure breathlessness in palliative care? A systematic review. Palliat Med. 2007;21:177–91.

27. Jennings AL, Davies AN, Higgins JPT, et al. A systematic review of the use of opioids in the management of dyspnoea. Thorax. 2002;57:939–44.

28. Simon ST, Higginson IJ, Booth S, et al. Benzodiazepines for the relief of breathlessness in advanced malignant and non-malignant diseases in adults. Cochrane Database Syst Rev. 2010;(1):CD 007354.

29. Booth S, Anderson H, Swannick M, et al. The use of oxygen in the palliation of breathless-ness. A report of the expert working group of the scientific committee of the association of palliative medicine. Respir Med. 2003;98:66–77.

30. Bredin M, Corner J, Krishnasamy M, et al. Multicentre randomised controlled trial of nursing intervention for breathlessness in patients with lung cancer. BMJ. 1999;318:901–4.

31. Sachs S, Weinberg RL. Pulmonary rehabilitation for dyspnea in the palliative-care setting. Curr Opin Support Palliat Care. 2009;3:112–9.

32. Fallon M, O'Neill B. ABC of palliative care. Constipation and diarrhoea. BMJ. 1997;315:1293–6.

33. Clemens K, Klaschik E. Managing opioid-induced constipation in advanced illness: focus on methylnaltrexone bromide. Ther Clin Risk Manag. 2010;6:77–82.

34. Sykes N. Constipation and diarrhoea. In: Hanks G, Cherny N, Kaasa S, editors. Oxford textbook of palliative medicine. 4th ed. Oxford: Oxford University Press; 2010. p. 833–50.

35. Rentz AM, van Hanswijck de Jonge P, Leyendecker P, Hopp M. Observational, noninterven-tion, multicenter study for validation of the Bowel Function Index for constipation in European countries. Curr Med Res Opin. 2011;27:35–44.

36. Larkin PJ, Sykes NP, Centeno C, et al. The management of constipation in palliative care: clinical practice recommendations. Palliat Med. 2008;22:796–807.

37. Thomas J, Karver S, Cooney GA, et al. Methylnaltrexone for opioid-induced constipation in advanced illness. N Engl J Med. 2008;358:2332–43.

38. Piirilä P, Sovijärvi AR. Objective assessment of cough. Eur Respir J. 1995;8:1949–56.

39. Symptom management. In: Watson M, Lucas C, Hoy A, Back I, editors. Oxford handbook of palliative care. Oxford: Oxford University Press; 2005:363–380.

40. Irwin RS, French CT, Fletcher KE. Quality of life in coughers. Pulm Pharmacol Ther. 2002;15:283–6.

41. Molassiotis A, Smith JA, Bennett MI, et al. Clinical expert guidelines for the management of cough in lung cancer: report of a UK task group on cough. Cough. 2010;6:9.

42. Birring SS, Prudon B, Carr AJ, et al. Development of a symptom specific health status measure for patients with chronic cough: Leicester Cough Questionnaire (LCQ). Thorax. 2003;58:339–43.

43. French CT, Irwin RS, Fletcher KE, Adams TM. Evaluation of a cough-specific quality-of-life questionnaire. Chest. 2002;121:1123–31.

44. Wee B. Chronic cough. Curr Opin Support Palliat Care. 2008;2:105–9.

45. Bonneau A. Cough in the palliative care setting. Can Fam Physician. 2009;55:600–2.

46. Estfan B, LeGrand S. Management of cough in advanced cancer. J Support Oncol. 2004;2:523–7.

47. Davis C, Percy G. Breathlessness, cough, and other respiratory symptoms. In: Fallon M, Hanks G, editors. ABC of palliative care. 2nd ed. Oxford: Blackwell Publishing; 2006. p. 13–6.

48. NHS Scotland. Delirium. 2009. Available at: www.palliativecareguidelines.scot.nhs.uk/documents/Delirium.pdf. Last accessed 27 Nov 2011.

49. Alici Y, Breibart W. Delirium in palliative care. Prim Psychiatry. 2009;16:42–8.

50. National Institute for Health and Clinical Excellence. Delirium. Diagnosis, prevention and management. NICE clinical guidelines 103. London: National Clinical Guideline Centre for Acute and Chronic Conditions; 2010.

51. Leonard M, Raju B, Conroy M, et al. Reversibility of delirium in terminally ill patients and predictors of mortality. Palliat Med. 2008;22:848–54.

52. Centeno C, Sanz A, Bruera E. Delirium in advanced cancer patients. Palliat Med. 2004;18:184–94.

53. Cohen MZ, Pace EA, Kaur G, Bruera E. Delirium in advanced cancer leading to distress in patients and family caregivers. J Palliat Care. 2009;25:164–71.

54. Palliative Drugs. Essential independent drug information for palliative and hospice care. Formulary 2011. Available at: www.palliativedrugs.com. Last accessed 27 Nov 2011.

55. Cherny NI, Radbruch L, Board of the European Association for Palliative Care. European Association for Palliative Care (EAPC) recommended framework for the use of sedation in palliative care. Palliat Med. 2009;23:581–93.

56. World Health Organization. Mental health: depression. 2011. Available at: www.who.int/mental_health/management/depression/definition/en. Last accessed 27 Nov 2011.

57. Noorani NH, Mantagnini M. Recognizing depression in palliative care patients. J Palliat Med. 2007;10:458–64.

58. Block SD. Assessing and managing depression in the terminally ill patient. ACP-ASIM End-of-Life Care Consensus Panel. American College of Physicians – American Society of Internal Medicine. Ann Intern Med. 2000;132:209–18.

59. Chochinov HM, Wilson KG, Enns M, et al. Desire for death in the terminally ill. Am J Psychiatry. 1995;152:1185–91.

60. Montano CB. Recognition and treatment of depression in a primary care setting. J Clin Psychiatry. 1994;55 suppl 12:S18–34.

61. Ellen SR, Norman TR, Burrows GD. MJA practice essentials. 3. Assessment of anxiety and depression in primary care. Med J Aust. 1997;167:328–33.

62. Rayner L, Higginson IJ, Price A, Hotopf M. The management of depression in palliative care: draft European clinical guidelines. London: Department of Palliative Care, Policy & Rehabilitation/European Palliative Care Research Collaborative; 2009.

63. Rayner L, Loge JH, Wasteson E, Higgson IJ. The detection of depression in palliative care. Curr Opin Support Palliat Care. 2009;3:55–60.

64. Price A, Hotopf M. The treatment of depression in patients with advanced cancer undergoing palliative care. Curr Opin Support Palliat Care. 2009;3:61–6.

65. Wilkinson SM, Love SB, Westcombe AM, et al. Effectiveness of aromatherapy massage in the management of anxiety and depression in patients with cancer: a multicenter randomized controlled trial. J Clin Oncol. 2007;25:532–9.

66. National institute for Health and Clinical Excellence. Depression with a chronic physical health problem: full guideline CG91. 2009. Available at: www.nice.org.uk/nicemedia/live/12327/45913/45913.pdf. Last accessed 27 Nov 2011.

67. Sykes N, Ripamonti C, Bruera E, Gordon D. Constipation, diarrhoea and intestinal obstruction. In: Fallon M, Hanks G, editors. ABC of palliative care. 2nd ed. Oxford: Blackwell Publishing; 2006. p. 29–35.

68. Dalal S, Bruera E. Dehydration in cancer patients: to treat or not to treat. J Support Oncol. 2004;2:467–79.

69. Davies AN. Oral symptoms. In: Sykes N, Edmonds P, Wiles J, editors. Management of advanced disease. 4th ed. London: Arnold; 2006. p. 168–74.

70. Lew J, Smith JA. Mucosal graft-vs-host disease. Oral Dis. 2007;13:519–29.

71. Bhide SA, Miah AB, Harrington KJ, Newbold KL, Nutting CM. Radiation-induced xerostomia: pathophysiology, prevention and treatment. Clin Oncol. 2009;21:737–44.

72. De Conno F, Martini C, Sbanotto A, Ripamonti C, Ventafridda V. Mouth care. In: Hanks G, Cherny N, Kaasa S, et al., editors. Oxford textbook of palliative medicine. 4th ed. Oxford: Oxford University Press; 2010. p. 996–1014.

73. World Gastroenterology Organisation. Practice guidelines. Dysphagia. 2007. Available at: www.worldgastroenterology.org/assets/downloads/en/pdf/guidelines/08_dysphagia.pdf. Last accessed 27 Nov 2011.

74. Swann D, Edmonds P. Dysphagia. In: Sykes N, Edmonds P, Wiles J, editors. Management of advanced disease. 4th ed. London: Arnold; 2006. p. 136–45.

75. Regnard C. Dysphagia, dyspepsia and hiccup. In: Hanks G, Cherny N, Kaasa S, et al., editors. Oxford textbook of palliative medicine. 4th ed. Oxford: Oxford University Press; 2010. p. 812–33.

76. Porter SR, Scully C. Oral malodour (halitosis). BMJ. 2006;333:632–5.

77. van den Broek AM, Feenstra L, de Baat C. A review of the current literature on aetiology and measurement methods of halitosis. J Dent. 2007;35:627–35.

78. Yaegaki K, Coil JM. Examination, classification and treatment of halitosis: clinical perspectives. J Can Dent Assoc. 2000;66:257–61.

79. Bagg J, Davies A. Oral health in patients with advanced disease. In: Fallon M, Hanks G, editors. ABC of palliative care. 2nd ed. Oxford: Blackwell Publishing; 2006. p. 17–20.

80. Krakauer EL, Zhu AX, Bounds BC, et al. Case 6–2005. A 58-year-old man with oesophageal cancer and nausea, vomiting, and intractable hiccups. N Engl J Med. 2005;352:817–25.

81. Perdue C, Lloyd E. Managing persistent hiccups in advanced cancer 1: physiology. Nurs Times. 2008;104:24–5.

82. Perdue C, Lloyd E. Managing persistent hiccups in advanced cancer 2: treatment. Nurs Times. 2008;104:20–1.

83. Hardy J. The treatment of hiccups in terminal patients. Eur J Palliat Care. 2003;10:192–3.

84. Malone M, Harris AL, Luscombe DK. Assessment of the impact of cancer on work, recreation, home management and sleep using a general health status measure. J R Soc Med. 1994;87:386–9.

85. Mercadante S, Girelli D, Casuccio A. Sleep disorders in advanced cancer patients: prevalence and factors associated. Supp Care Cancer. 2004;12:355–9.

86. Davidson JR, MacLean AW, Brundage MD, Schulze K. Sleep disturbances in cancer patients. Soc Sci Med. 2002;54:1309–21.

87. Sateia MJ, Byock IR. Sleep in palliative care. In: Hanks G, Cherny N, Kaasa S, et al., editors. Oxford textbook of palliative medicine. 4th ed. Oxford: Oxford University Press; 2010. p. 1059–83.

88. Hugel H, Ellershaw JE, Cook L, et al. The prevalence, key causes and management of insomnia in palliative care patients. J Pain Symptom Manage. 2004;27:316–21.

89. Sarris J, Byrne GJ. A systematic review of insomnia and complementary medicine. Sleep Med Rev. 2011;15:99–106.

90. Savard J, Simard S, Ivers H, et al. Randomized study on the efficacy of cognitive – behavioral therapy for insomnia: part I: sleep and psychological effects. J Clin Oncol. 2005;23:6083–96.

91. Waller A, Caroline NL. Handbook of palliative care in cancer. Woburn: Butterworth-Heinemann; 2000. p. 115–24.

92. Zylicz Z, Krajnik M. Pruritus in the course of malignancy. In: Misery L, Ständer S, editors. Pruritus. London: Springer; 2010.

93. Twycross R, Greaves MW, Handwerker H, et al. Itch: scratching more than the surface. Q J Med. 2003;96:7–26.

94. Pittelkow MR, Loprinzi CL. Pruritus and sweating in palliative medicine. In: Hanks G, Cherny N, Kaasa S, et al., editors. Oxford textbook of palliative medicine. 4th ed. Oxford: Oxford University Press; 2010. p. 934–51.

95. Borup Christensen S, Lundgren E. Sequelae of axillary dissection vs. axillary sampling with or without irradiation for breast cancer. A randomized trial. Acta Chir Scand. 1989;155:515–9.

96. Moffat CJ, Franks PJ, Doherty DC, et al. Lymphoedema: an underestimated health problem. Q J Med. 2003;96:731–8.

97. International Society of Lymphology. Consensus document. The diagnosis and treatment of peripheral lymphedema. Lymphology. 2003;36:84–91.

98. Williams AF, Franks PJ, Moffat CJ. Lymphoedema: estimating the size of the problem. Palliat Med. 2005;19:300–13.

99. Keeley V. Lymphoedema. In: Hanks G, Cherny N, Kaasa S, et al., editors. Oxford textbook of palliative medicine. 4th ed. Oxford: Oxford University Press; 2010. p. 972–82.

100. Engel J, Kerr J, Schlesinger-Raab A, et al. Predictors of quality of life of breast cancer patients. Acta Oncol. 2003;42:710–8.

101. Sitzia J, Sobrido L. Measurement of health-related quality of life of patients receiving conservative treatment for limb lymphoedema using the Nottingham Health Profile. Qual Life Res. 1997;6:373–84.

102. Badger C, Preston NJ, Seers K, Mortimer P. Benzo-pyrones for reducing and controlling lymphoedema of the limbs. Cochrane Database Syst Rev. 2004;(2):CD003140.

103. Ripamonti CI, Easson AM, Gerdes H. Management of malignant bowel obstruction. Eur J Cancer. 2008;44:1105–15.

104. Downing GM. Bowel obstruction. In: Downing GM, Wainwright W, editors. Medical care of the dying. 4th ed. Victoria: Victoria Hospice Society Learning Centre for Palliative Care; 2006. p. 333–9.

105. Letizia M, Norton E. Successful management of malignant bowel obstruction. J Hosp Palliat Nurs. 2003;5:152–8.

106. Edmonds P, Wiles J. Pleural effusions. In: Sykes N, Edmonds P, Wiles J, editors. Management of advanced disease. 4th ed. London: Arnold; 2006. p. 289–93.

107. Musani AI. Treatment options for malignant pleural effusion. Curr Opin Pulm Med. 2009;15:380–7.

108. Roberts ME, Neville E, Berrisford RG, Antunes G, Ali NJ. Management of a malignant pleural effusion: British Thoracic Society Pleural Disease Guideline 2010. Thorax. 2010;65 suppl 2:ii32–40.

109. Woodruff R. Palliative medicine. 4th ed. Melbourne: Oxford University Press; 2004.

110. Moffett PU, Moffett BK, Laber DA. Diagnosing and managing suspected malignant pleural effusions. J Support Oncol. 2009;7:143–6.

111. Maida V, Ennis M, Kuziemsky C, Trozzolo L. Symptoms associated with malignant wounds: a prospective case series. J Pain Symptom Manage. 2009;37:206–11.

112. Naylor W. Malignant wounds: aetiology and principles of management. Nurs Stand. 2002;16:45–56.

113. McDonald A, Lesage P. Palliative management of pressure ulcers and malignant wounds in patients with advanced illness. J Palliat Med. 2006;9:285–95.

114. World Health Organization. Cancer pain relief. 2nd ed. Geneva: WHO; 1996.

115. Zeppetella G. Topical opioids for painful skin ulcers: does it work? Eur J Palliat Care. 2004;11:93–6.

116. Morgan D. Wounds – what should a dressing formulary include? Hosp Pharm. 2002;9:261–6.

117. Grocott P. Care of patients with fungating malignant wounds. Nurs Stand. 2007;21:57–66.

118. Wilson V. Assessment and management of fungating wounds: a review. Br J Commun Nurs. 2005;10 suppl 3:S28–34.

119. Grocott P, Robinson V. Skin problems in palliative care – nursing perspective. In: Hanks G, Cherny N, Kaasa S, et al., editors. Oxford textbook of palliative medicine. 4th ed. Oxford: Oxford University Press; 2010. p. 961–72.

120. Potter JM, Reid DB, Shaw RJ, et al. Myoclonus associated with treatment with high doses of morphine: the role of supplemental drugs. BMJ. 1989;299:150–3.

121. Sweeney C, Bruera ED. Opioid side effects and management. In: Bruera ED, Porternoy RK, editors. Cancer pain assessment and management. Cambridge: Cambridge University Press; 2003. p. 150–70.

122. Rhodes VA, McDaniel RW. Nausea, vomiting, and retching: complex problems in palliative care. CA Cancer J Clin. 2001;51:232–48.

123. Vainio A, Auvinen A. Symptom Prevalence Group. Prevalence of symptoms among patients with advanced cancer: an international collaborative study. J Pain Symptom Manage. 1996;12:3–10.

124. Fainsinger R, Miller MJ, Bruera E, et al. Symptom control during the last week of life on a palliative care unit. J Palliat Care. 1991;7:5–11.

125. Mannix K. Nausea and vomiting. In: Fallon M, Hanks G, editors. ABC of palliative care. 2nd ed. Oxford: Blackwell Publishing; 2006. p. 25–8.

126. Patient UK. Nausea and vomiting in palliative care. 2011. Available at: www.patient.co.uk/doctor/Nausea-and-Vomiting-in-Palliative-Care.htm. Last accessed 27 Nov 2011.

127. Twycross R. Anorexia, cachexia, nausea and vomiting. Medicine. 2004;32:9–13.

128. van den Beuken-van Everdingen MH, de Rijke JM, Kessels AG, et al. Prevalence of pain in patients with cancer: a systematic review of the past 40 years. Ann Oncol. 2007;18: 1437–49.

129. Twycross R, Lack S. Symptom control in far advanced cancer. London: Pitman; 1983.

130. Diagnosing neuropathic pain in clinical practice. In: Bennett MI, editor. Neuropathic pain. Oxford: Oxford University Press; 2006:25–35.

131. Bennett M. The LANSS pain scale: the Leeds assessment of neuropathic symptoms and signs. Pain. 2001;92:147–57.

132. Levy MH. Pharmacologic treatment of cancer pain. N Engl J Med. 1996;335:1124–32.

133. Hanks GW, De Conno F, Cherny N, et al. Morphine and alternative opioids in cancer pain: the EAPC recommendations. Br J Cancer. 2001;84:587–93.

134. Scottish Intercollegiate Guidelines Network. Control of pain in adults with cancer. A national clinical guideline. Edinburgh: SIGN; 2008.

135. Zeppetella G. Alternative routes for opioid administration. In: Forbes K, editor. Opioids for cancer pain. Oxford: Oxford University Press; 2007. p. 101–9.

136. Palliative Drugs. Buprenorphine. Available at: www.palliativedrugs.com/buprenorphine.html. Last accessed 27 Nov 2011.

137. Cherny N, Ripamonti C, Pereira J, et al. Strategies to manage the adverse effects of oral morphine: an evidence-based report. J Clin Oncol. 2001;19:2542–54.

138. Fallon M, Hanks G, Charney N. Principles of control of cancer pain. In: Fallon M, Hanks G, editors. ABC of palliative care. 2nd ed. Oxford: Blackwell Publishing; 2006. p. 4–7.

139. Cleeland CS, Ryan KM. Pain assessment: global use of the Brief Pain Inventory. Ann Acad Med Singapore. 1994;23:129–38.

140. Zeppetella G, Bates C. Scientific evidence and expert clinical opinion for the clinical utility of opioid switching. In: Hillier R, Finlay I, Miles A, editors. The effective management of cancer pain. 2nd ed. London: Aesculapius Medical Press; 2002. p. 39–55.

141. International Association for the Study of Pain. Barriers to cancer pain treatment. 2009. Available at: www.iasp-pain.org/AM/Template.cfm?Section=Home&Template=/CM/ContentDisplay.cfm&ContentID=7189. Last accessed 27 Nov 2011.

142. MIMS. Monthly Index of Medical Specialities. Available at: www.mims.co.uk/Tables/940779/Co-Analgesics-Use-Cancer-Pain. Last accessed 27 Nov 2011.

143. Kohn M. The State of CAM in UK cancer care: advances in research, practice and delivery. Available at: www.cancer.gov/cam/attachments/cam-in-uk-summary.pdf. Last accessed 27 Nov 2011.

144. Davies AN, Dickman A, Reid C, et al. The management of cancer-related breakthrough pain: recommendations of a task group of the Science Committee of the Association for Palliative Medicine of Great Britain and Ireland. Eur J Pain. 2009;13:331–8.

145. Zeppetella G, Ribeiro MD. The pharmacotherapy of cancer-related episodic pain. Expert Opin Pharmacother. 2003;4:493–502.

146. Zeppetella G. Impact and management of breakthrough pain in cancer. Curr Opin Support Palliat Care. 2009;3:1–6.

147. Zeppetella G. Oral transmucosal opioid drugs. In: Davies A, editor. Cancer-related breakthrough pain. Oxford: Oxford University Press; 2006. p. 57–71.

148. Zeppetella G. Successful management of breakthrough pain in cancer patients. London: Evolving Medicine Ltd; 2011.

149. Davies A. General principles of management. In: Davies A, editor. Cancer-related breakthrough pain. Oxford: Oxford University Press; 2006. p. 31–42.

150. Daniel WJ. Anorectal pain, bleeding and lumps. Aust Fam Physician. 2010;39:376–81.

151. Mercadante S, Fulfaro F, Dabbene M. Methadone in treatment of tenesmus not responding to morphine escalation. Support Care Cancer. 2001;9:129–30.

152. Sonis ST, Eilers JP, Epstein JB, et al. Validation of a new scoring system for the assessment of clinical trial research of oral mucositis induced by radiation or chemotherapy. Mucositis Study Group. Cancer. 1999;85:2103–13.

153. McGuire DB, Altomonte V, Peterson DE, et al. Patterns of mucositis and pain in patients receiving preparative chemotherapy and bone marrow transplantation. Oncol Nurs Forum. 1993;20:1493–502.

154. Brown CG, Yoder LH. Stomatitis: an overview. Am J Nurs. 2002;102 suppl 4:20–3.

155. World Health Organization. WHO handbook for reporting results of cancer treatment. Geneva: World Health Organization; 1979.

156. Worthington HV, Clarkson JE, Bryan G, et al. Interventions for preventing oral mucositis for patients with cancer receiving treatment. Cochrane Database Syst Rev. 2010;(12):CD000978.

157. Vayne-Bossert P, Escher M, de Vautibault CG, et al. Effect of topical morphine (mouthwash) on oral pain due to chemotherapy- and/or radiotherapy-induced mucositis: a randomized double-blinded study. J Palliat Med. 2010;13:125–8.

158. Clarkson JE, Worthington HV, Furness S, et al. Interventions for treating oral mucositis for patients with cancer receiving treatment. Cochrane Database Syst Rev. 2010;(8):CD001973.

159. Swann D, Edmonds P. Sweating. In: Sykes N, Edmonds P, Wiles J, editors. Management of advanced disease. 4th ed. London: Arnold; 2006. p. 214–8.

160. Cheshire WP, Freeman R. Disorders of sweating. Semin Neurol. 2003;23:399–406.

161. Stolman LP. Treatment of hyperhidrosis. J Drugs Dermatol. 2003;2:521–7.

162. Murphy BA, Cmelak A, Bayles S, et al. Palliative issues in the care of patients with cancer of the head and neck. In: Hanks G, Cherny N, Kaasa S, et al., editors. Oxford textbook of palliative medicine. 4th ed. Oxford: Oxford University Press; 2010. p. 908–15.

163. Lichter I, Hunt E. The last 48 hours of life. J Palliat Care. 1990;6:7–15.

164. Harris A. Providing urinary continence care to adults at the end of life. Nurs Times. 2009;105:29.

165. Swann D, Edmonds P. The management of urinary symptoms. In: Sykes N, Edmonds P, Wiles J, editors. Management of advanced disease. 4th ed. London: Arnold; 2006. p. 219–24.

166. Gerber LH, Stout N. Factors predicting clinically significant fatigue in women following treatment for primary breast cancer. Support Care Cancer. 2011;19:1581–91.

167. NHS Scotland. Fatigue. Available at: www.palliativecareguidelines.scot.nhs.uk/documents/Fatigue.pdf. Last accessed 27 Nov 2011.

168. Mock V. Fatigue management. Evidence and guidelines for practice. Cancer. 2001;92:1699–707.

Chapter 5

Palliative Care Emergencies

Patients receiving palliative care may deteriorate suddenly due to their illness or another acute medical or surgical problem. Management options depend on life expectancy, level of intervention needed, and an assessment of risks, benefits, side effects, and likely outcome.

Emergencies may be completely unexpected, but some can be predicted from the nature and location of the patient's disease (e.g., SCC in patients with vertebral metastases, bowel obstruction in patients with peritoneal disease, or bleeding in patients with tumors encroaching on large vessels or who have bone marrow failure). Emergencies can also include a sudden severe exacerbation of symptoms; these are described elsewhere.

The distinction to be made is whether the patient is unwell because of overall progression in (maximally) treated disease or because of the effects of an acute problem with an easily reversible cause.

Assessment

Palliative care emergencies should be assessed based on the following [1]:

- the nature of the emergency,
- the patient's general physical condition,
- disease status and likely prognosis,
- concomitant pathologies,
- symptoms,
- benefits versus risks, and
- patients' and carers' wishes.

G. Zeppetella, *Palliative Care in Clinical Practice*,
DOI 10.1007/978-1-4471-2843-4_5,
© Springer-Verlag London 2012

Important considerations to take into account:
- the life-limiting illness,
- intercurrent illness,
- response to disease or prognosis-modifying therapies,
- change in functional status over time, and
- the patient's perception of their future.

Advance care planning (ACP):
- anticipate,
- advance care plan,
- does patient want resuscitation?
- is admission appropriate?

The drugs most frequently used in an emergency are:
- morphine injection 10 or 20 mg ampoule,
- midazolam injection 5 mg/mL – 2 mL ampoule for subcutaneous or buccal administration,
- lorazepam 1 mg tablet for sublingual (prescribed as Genus brand) or oral use,
- haloperidol injection 5 mg/mL ampoule for subcutaneous administration,
- glycopyrronium injection 200 µg/mL – 1 mL ampoule for subcutaneous administration, and
- water for injection.

Systems are required to ensure that palliative care patients have prompt and easy access to appropriate medicines, particularly during the 'out-of-hours' period. 'Just in case' boxes are used in some primary care trusts in the UK, where a predetermined list of drugs can be ordered and used in emergencies or at the end of life. The boxes are provided with written instructions for the supply or administration of medicines to patients who may not be individually identified before presentation for treatment, so-called 'patient group directions'.

The next section provides a brief summary of emergencies commonly seen in a palliative care setting.

Hemorrhage
Definition
Hemorrhage is the flow of blood from a ruptured blood vessel.

Prevalence
Metastatic malignancy increases the risk of bleeding and thrombosis, and approximately 6–14% of patients with cancer have bleeds. In 3–12% of patients, bleeding contributes to death [2]. Massive hemorrhage is rare.

Assessment
Hemorrhage may be caused by trauma, ulceration, inflammation, or a growth that erodes through a blood vessel (Figure 5.1). Hemorrhage usually occurs at the site of the malignancy. The carotid artery, femoral artery, and intrapulmonary vessels are reported to be the most common sites [2]. Bleeding can be external or internal and predisposing factors include the following:

- cancer-related: abnormal clotting, platelet dysfunction,
- chemotherapy-related: reduced platelet count,
- biochemical: uremia, hepatic dysfunction,
- pharmacological: NSAIDs, anticoagulants, and
- tumor invasion: hemoptysis, gastrointestinal bleed.

Causes of hemorrhage in palliative care patient	
ENT tumor	Carotid artery erosion from neck metastases Oropharyngeal tumor erosion in mouth
Gastrointestinal hemorrhage	Gastroduodenal hematemesis Small or large bowel bleeding with melena
Bladder	Hematuria due to tumor, DIC, or leukemia
Leukemia or blood dyscrasia	Possible multiple sites, but external mouth or nasal bleeding is obviously distressing. Extensive ecchymoses are also visually difficult for many family members
DIC	Due to various causes such as sepsis
Other	Ruptured aortic aneurysm (or thoracic) Tumor lymph node erosion into adjacent vessels

Figure 5.1 Causes of hemorrhage in palliative care patients. *DIC* disseminated intravascular coagulation, *ENT* ear, nose, and throat

The bleeding may be visible or invisible, as in a gastrointestinal or other hemorrhage. Bleeding could be rapid (in the case of carotid artery erosion) or over several hours (when smaller vessels are affected).

Minor bleeding requires an assessment of whether the problem is local or systemic and routine investigations include CBC check, coagulation screen, and LFTs. With massive hemorrhage the patient is conscious for a short period of time (20 s to several minutes), before lapsing into a hypoxic coma followed by a cardiac arrest. It is not painful, but is often a terrifying experience for the patient and especially for the family and staff.

If a patient is having a large internal hemorrhage he or she is likely to exhibit most of the following:

- suddenly becoming tired and weak,
- pale, cold, clammy skin,
- sudden irritability and restlessness/panic,
- rapid heart rate and breathing, and
- loss of consciousness.

General Management

The possibility of hemorrhage can often be anticipated and a plan prepared. Certain cancers and conditions are more likely to be prone to hemorrhage and massive hemorrhage is often heralded by smaller bleeds.

Therapies predisposing to hemorrhage (e.g., aspirin, warfarin) should be stopped and the family prepared ahead of time or an explanation provided when an unexpected event occurs. Advanced planning is necessary for all patients with the potential to bleed, because this symptom is a source of considerable distress for patients, family, and staff (Figure 5.2) [2].

A major hemorrhage may be a terminal event and active treatment is not appropriate or possible. The following should be done:

- summon assistance,
- stay with the patient,
- if appropriate, wear gloves and other protective clothing,
- remain calm, talk quietly and reassuringly,
- keep the person warm with extra blankets,

Management of terminal hemorrhage in patients with advanced cancer

Identify patients at risk

General risk factors:
- Thrombocytopenia
- Large head and neck carcinomas
- Large centrally located lung cancers
- Refractory acute and chronic leukemia
- Myelodysplasia
- Metastatic liver desease and deranged clotting

Specific risk factors for carotid artery rupture:
- Surgery (eg, radical neck dissection)
- Radiotherapy
- Poor post-operative healing
- Visible arterial pulsation
- Pharyngo-cutaneous fistula
- Fungating tumors
- Systemic factors, eg, diabetes, age >50 years, 10–15% loss body weight, immunodeficiency, malnourishment

Multidisciplinary team discussion
- May include oncologist, surgeon, nursing staff, pharmacist, chaplain
- Proactive preparation and advance planning
- Factors to consider:
  - Patient's prognosis
  - Patient's performance status
  - Patient's perceived quality of life and preferences

Discussion with patient and family
- How likely the MDT feels that terminal hemorrhage may occur
- Patient and family's knowledge and acceptance of diagnosis and prognosis
- How much information the patient and carer want to receive
- Patient and family's desired level of participation in decisions about their care
- Patient and family's coping strategies

In event of hemorrhage, use measures to a level appropriate to the individual patient

General supportive measures, eg,:
- Call for assistance
- Ensure a nurse stays with the patient
- Provide psychological support
- Apply pressure if bleeding externally visible
- Use of dark towels to camouflage blood loss
- Use of suction if possible
- Use of sedative medication: currently no consensus regarding drug, dose, or route

General resuscitative measures, eg,:
- Volume and fluid replacement with colloid fluid or blood products

Specific intervention to stop the bleeding, eg,:
- Surgical ligation of an artery

After the event
- Debrief and support for relatives/carers and staff after the event
- Consider whether counseling is needed

Figure 5.2 Management of terminal hemorrhage in patients with advanced cancer. *MDT* multidisciplinary team. (Reproduced with permission from Harris and Noble [2])

- don't try to keep the person awake because this will only add to the stress of the situation,
- use dark-colored towels and linen to minimize the sight of blood,
- give medications, and
- ensure aftercare.

Pharmacological Management

There are a number of options for the pharmacological management of hemorrhage [3–5].

Small Bleeds
Topical Treatments
- Alginate dressings (redress as infrequently as possible),
- epinephrine: 1 in 10,000 (100 µg/mL), 10 mL ampoule, 1 mL, and 10 mL prefilled syringe, or 1 in 1,000 (1 mg/mL),
- tranexamic acid: 100 mg/mL in a 5 mL ampoule,
- silver nitrate: caustic pencil, tip containing silver nitrate 40%, potassium nitrate 60%, and
- sucralfate paste: 1 g tablets may be dispersed in water or suspension available of sucralfate, 1 g/5 mL.

Systemic Treatments
- Tranexamic acid (orally): 1–1.5 g bd/tds,
- etamsylate: 500 mg qds, and
- metronidazole: 400 mg tds.

Severe Hemorrhage
If the patient is distressed, titrated doses of a rapidly acting benzodiazepine are indicated. The route of administration guides the choice of drug:

- iv access available: midazolam 5–20 mg iv or diazepam (emulsion for intravenous injection) 5–20 mg iv in small boluses until settled,
- im injection: midazolam 5–10 mg im can be given into the deltoid muscle,
- rectal route or via a stoma: diazepam rectal solution 5–10 mg, or

- sublingual: midazolam 10 mg can be given using the parenteral preparation or the buccal liquid (unlicensed medicine; special order product).

Non-pharmacological Management

The non-pharmacological management of hemorrhage involves the following:

- radiotherapy,
- cryotherapy,
- laser,
- embolization, and
- surgery.

Bleeding that is external and severe is frightening and distressing for those witnessing it. After the event it is often valuable to offer a debriefing session to team members. Ongoing support should be provided as necessary for the relatives and staff.

Malignant Hypercalcemia
Definition

Malignant hypercalcemia is a corrected serum calcium of >2.6 mmol/L.

Prevalence

Of all patients with malignant disease 20% will develop hypercalcemia. Most commonly this occurs in breast, myeloma, renal cell and squamous cell tumors, and lymphoma [6].

Assessment

The clinical features of hypercalcemia are shown in Figure 5.3 [7]. Although neuromuscular, gastrointestinal, and renal manifestations are most common [8], symptoms may vary in individual patients and are related both to the absolute concentration of serum calcium and to the rate of rise in serum calcium:

$$\text{Corrected calcium}\,(\text{mmol}/\,L) = (40 \text{ serum albumin in g}/\,L) \times 0.02.$$

Symptoms associated with rising calcium	
Symptoms	Corrected calcium (mmol/L)
None or mild: fatigue, anorexia, nausea, constipation, polyuria	2.65–3.0
Moderate: vomiting, thirst, mild confusion, muscle weakness	3.0–3.5
Severe: dehydration, ileus, psychosis, drowsiness	3.5–4.0
Life threatening: bradyarrythmias, heart block, coma, systolic arrest, and death	>4.0

Figure 5.3 Symptoms associated with rising calcium. (Reproduced with permission from Bower and Cox [7])

For example, for a patient with a calcium of 2.45 mmol/L and albumin of 24 g/L:

$$\text{Corrected calcium} = [40 - 24] \times 0.02 = 2.77 \text{ mmol}/\text{L}.$$

Severe hypercalcemia is most likely the result of a vicious cycle. The hypercalcemic effects of anorexia, nausea, and vomiting along with impaired renal concentrating ability lead to dehydration and, subsequently, altered mental status. This, in turn, may promote immobilization and lead to worsening hypercalcemia [8].

In addition to the symptoms of hypercalcemia, the clinical features include signs and symptoms of the underlying cancer. Generally, the cancer is well advanced in patients when hypercalcemia occurs, and the prognosis is poor. Survival beyond 6 months is uncommon [9].

General Management

If hypercalcemia is suspected, first consider whether further intervention is appropriate or acceptable. If further intervention is required, admit the patient for rehydration and possible bisphosphonate therapy. For patients not undergoing interventional treatment, full symptomatic treatment should be continued.

The following are the initial goals of treatment:

- stabilization and reduction of the calcium level,
- adequate hydration,

- increased urinary calcium excretion,
- inhibition of osteoclast activity in the bone,
- discontinuation of pharmacological agents associated with hypercalcemia, and
- treatment of the underlying cause (when possible).

Pharmacological Management

There are a number of options for the pharmacological management of hypercalcemia [3–5].

Zoledronic Acid

Zoledronic acid (Zometa®) inhibits bone resorption, possibly by acting on osteoclasts or osteoclast precursors. The median duration of complete response (defined as maintaining normalized calcium levels) and the time to relapse is reported as 32 and 30 days, respectively [10]. Zoledronic acid is indicated for hypercalcemia of malignancy. The recommended dose is 4 mg intravenous infusion over at least a 15-min period each month, although the patient may be re-treated after 1 week if the desired response is not observed. The patient should be hydrated before infusion.

Pamidronate

Pamidronate (Aredia®) works by inhibiting normal and abnormal bone resorption. It appears to inhibit bone resorption without inhibiting bone formation and mineralization. The adverse effects associated with intravenous administration include mild transient increases in temperature, leukopenia, and a mild reduction in serum phosphate levels. The recommended dose in moderate hypercalcemia is a 60-mg intravenous infusion over 4 h initially. Alternatively, a 90-mg intravenous infusion should be administered over 24 h initially. In cases of severe hypercalcemia a 90-mg intravenous infusion should be given over 24 h initially.

Ibandronic Acid

Ibandronic acid (Bondronat®, Bonviva®) inhibits bone resorption by inhibiting the action of the osteoclasts. The reduction of bone loss helps prevent fractures in patients with bone metastases and reduces the amount of calcium released into the blood. The recommended dose by intravenous infusion, according to the serum calcium concentration, is 2–4 mg in a single infusion. The oral dose for Bondronat tablets is 50 mg/day or, for Bonviva tablets, 150 mg/month. The tablets should be swallowed whole with plenty of water while sitting or standing. They should be taken on an empty stomach at least 30 min (Bondronat) or 1 h (Bonviva) before the first food or drink (other than water) of the day, or another oral medicine. The patient should stand or sit upright for at least 1 h after taking the tablet.

It is strongly recommended that a dental check-up is considered before initiating bisphosphonate due to risk of osteonecrosis of the jaw.

The Medicines and Healthcare products Regulatory Agency and the Commission on Human Medicines advice on bisphosphonates and osteonecrosis of the jaw [3]:

- The risk of osteonecrosis of the jaw is substantially greater for patients receiving intravenous bisphosphonates in the treatment of cancer than for patients receiving oral bisphosphonates for osteoporosis or Paget's disease.
- Risk factors for developing osteonecrosis of the jaw that should be considered are: potency of bisphosphonate (highest for zolendronate), route of administration, cumulative dose, duration and type of malignant disease, concomitant treatment, smoking, comorbid conditions, and history of dental disease.
- All patients receiving bisphosphonates for cancer should have a dental check-up (and any necessary remedial work should be performed) before bisphosphonate treatment. However, urgent bisphosphonate treatment should not be delayed, and a dental check-up should be carried out as soon as possible in these patients. All other patients who are prescribed bisphosphonates should have a dental examination only if they have poor dental health.
- During bisphosphonate treatment patients should maintain good oral hygiene, receive routine dental check-ups, and report any oral symptoms.

Calcitonin

Calcitonin (Miacalcin®, Cibacalcin®, Calcimar®) is a naturally occurring hormone that inhibits bone absorption and increases the excretion of calcium. The effects of calcitonin may be observed within a few hours, with a peak response observed at 12–24 h. As a result of its short duration of action, other more potent but slower-acting agents should be used in patients with severe hypercalcemia. Salmon calcitonin is used most often and is more potent than human calcitonin. The action of this agent is short-lived. If there is a severe elevation of calcium, coadminister one to two doses with fluids and furosemide to provide a rapid, although limited, reduction of the calcium level. The recommended dose of calcitonin is 2–8 U/kg im/sc q6–12h.

Gallium Nitrate

Gallium nitrate (Ganite®) works by inhibiting bone reabsorption and altering the structure of bone crystals. It exerts a hypocalcemic effect, possibly by reducing bone resorption. Although gallium nitrate performs well against other anti-calcium agents, it has slow onset of action. The recommended dose of gallium nitrate in severe hypercalcemia is 200 mg/m²/day iv for 5 days in 1 L 0.9% saline. In cases of mild hypercalcemia, the recommended dose is 100 mg/m²/day iv for 5 days in 1 L 0.9% saline.

Corticosteroids

Although corticosteroids do not treat hypercalcemia, directly, they are useful for treating hypercalcemia caused by vitamin D toxicity, certain malignancies (e.g., multiple myeloma, lymphoma), sarcoidosis, and other granulomatous diseases. These agents are generally not effective in patients with solid tumors or primary hyperparathyroidism. Several different glucocorticoids may be used. The recommended dose of hydrocortisone is 200–300 mg iv for 3 days.

Resistant Hypercalcemia

Of patients presenting with hypercalcemia 80% survive less than 1 year [11]. If at assessment it is thought that the patient is dying or previous treatment had not led to a fall in serum calcium, palliation of symptoms (e.g., delirium, nausea, and pain) is required.

Malignant Spinal Cord Compression
Definition

Malignant SCC is the exertion of an abnormal amount of pressure on the spinal cord by a tumor (Figure 5.4).

Prevalence

SCC occurs in up to 5–10% of cancer patients and the incidence depends on the type of primary cancer, the most common being breast, prostate, and lung cancers [12, 13]. Approximately 10% of compressions occur at the cervical level of the spine, 70% at the thoracic level, and 20% at the lumbosacral level; there may be more than one site or level of compression [1].

Assessment

The symptoms and signs of SCC are variable, and so the most important factor in assessing patients is to have a high index of suspicion, with the

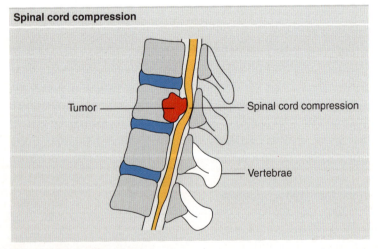

Figure 5.4 Spinal cord compression

Neurological signs and symptoms in spinal cord compression	
Symptoms	**Neurological signs and site**
Weak shoulders/upper limbs or hands/fingers	Cervical cord lesion: may be associated with symptoms/signs in legs or urinary dysfunction
Neck pain or pain radiating from shoulders to arm or fingers	Weakness/sensory signs in upper limbs. Increased tone in legs. Extensor plantar responses
Difficulty walking Stumbling over kerbs or steps	Thoracic cord lesion: may be associated with hesitancy of urine or retention or constipation
Unable to climb stairs Difficulty walking	Upper motor neuron weakness in legs (increased tone flexors weaker than extensors) with increased knee and ankle jerks, and extensor plantars
Paresthesia in lower limbs and buttocks Thoracic back pain	Sensory level with reduced sensation below level of compression: as a guide umbilicus is T10 (see Appendix 2)
Loss of bladder/bowel sensation	Cauda equina compression
Urinary retention often painless	Reduced tone in lower limbs, global weakness
Leg weakness	Reduced/absent knee and ankle jerks
Paresthesia/nerve pain in legs or buttocks	Flexor plantar responses
Low back pain	Sensory loss in lumbosacral dermatomes (ie, groins/legs and buttocks)

Figure 5.5 Neurological signs and symptoms in spinal cord compression

aim of diagnosing the problem when there are symptoms, but before the patient develops progressive neurological signs, because this affords him or her the best chance of remaining ambulatory. To wait for signs is possibly to leave it too late (Figure 5.5).

More than 25% of patients develop paraplegia within less than 48 h from presentation. Delays in diagnosis and treatment lead to a poorer outcome for the patient, with an increased risk of permanent disability and dependence. Fewer than 10% of patients unable to walk at diagnosis are likely to regain full mobility [14].

General Management

In cases of suspected SCC, there needs to be an urgent discussion with the oncologist and admission of the patient for MRI and treatment. Once SCC has been confirmed, definitive treatment should be given without delay, ideally within 24 h of onset of symptoms.

Factors influencing the decision-making process	
Patient factors	Prognosis Fitness for the planned surgery/comorbidities Age and functional status
General tumor factors	Tumor type, behavior, and radiosensitivity Number and site of extraspinal metastases
Local tumor factors	Pathoanatomy Number of spinal levels involved
Clinical problem	Neurological status (deficit and progression including speed) Pain Instability (actual or imminent)

Figure 5.6 **Factors influencing the decision-making process**. (Data from Akram and Allibone [15]. © 2010, with permission from Elsevier)

There may be occasional patients for whom hospice admission would be appropriate (e.g., end-stage disease, not fit for radiotherapy), but these should be discussed with the hospice medical staff on an individual basis. The factors that will influence the decision are listed in Figure 5.6 [15].

Pharmacological Management

The pharmacological management of SCC is as follows [16]:

- Dexamethasone 16 mg/day (unless there are specific contraindications), given orally if possible (but can be given subcutaneously or intravenously if necessary).
- Analgesia according to the patient's current therapy.
- Bisphosphonates to reduce pain and the risk of vertebral fracture/collapse may be of help in patients with vertebral involvement from myeloma or breast cancer.

Non-pharmacological Management

The non-pharmacological approaches to the management of SCC are as follows [17, 18]:

- Radiotherapy is the most common treatment for SCC in cancer patients. It can be used following decompression operations or used alone.
- Surgery is quite limited in advanced cancer patients and only suitable for those with a life expectancy longer than 3 months and with favorable performance status, whose tumor is not

radiosensitive. Where there is spinal stability a neurosurgical referral is required with a view to stabilization.

- Chemotherapy may be considered alongside other treatment modalities in patients with chemosensitive tumors and early signs of compression.
- Physiotherapy and rehabilitation is an essential part of management because median survival after compression and resultant impairment is 7–10 months, although up to 30% of patients live for more than 1 year.

Neutropenic Sepsis
Definition
Neutropenic sepsis is defined as follows:

- temperature ≥38°C on at least one occasion,
- neutrophil count adults: $<0.5 \times 10^9$/L (isolation, nursing, and dietary protocols for neutropenic patients generally apply to patients with neutrophils $<0.5 \times 10^9$/L),
- hypotension and/or tachycardia, and
- recent chemotherapy administration (within the previous 14 days).

Prevalence
Neutropenic sepsis is a recognized and potentially fatal complication of anticancer treatment (particularly chemotherapy), although there are no accurate data available for morbidity and mortality in adults. For example, mortality rates have variously been reported as between 2% and 21% [19].

Assessment
Neutropenic sepsis largely affects patients undergoing chemotherapy in whom the bone marrow is suppressed, and tends to present as a dip in the number of white cells (especially neutrophils), at approximately 10–15 days after treatment. The risk factors for developing neutropenic sepsis are shown in Figure 5.7.

The key features of neutropenic sepsis are:

- chemotherapy within the last 2 weeks,
- general flu-like symptoms with chills,

Risk factors for developing neutropenic sepsis induced by chemotherapy

Patient characteristics	Comorbid diseases, eg, cardiovascular or renal disease Older age, especially patients age >65 years Poor performance status Poor nutrition status Female sex Body surface area <2m^2 Previous episodes of neutropenic sepsis
Laboratory investigations	Hb <12g/dL Pretreatment absolute neutrophil count <1.5 × 10^9/L Low serum albumin
Disease characteristics	Cytopenias due to bone marrow infiltration by tumor Advanced cancer
Treatment	Myelotoxicity of the chemotherapy regimen Combined chemotherapy and radiotherapy Extensive prior treatment including radiation field No granulocyte-stimulating factor used

Figure 5.7 Risk factors for developing neutropenic sepsis induced by chemotherapy

- temperature >38°C,
- may be an obvious focus of infection, e.g., chest or urine infection, and
- where a recent blood count is known, a neutrophil count <1.0 × 10^9/L makes sepsis more likely.

Assessment will depend upon the clinical setting and can include the following:
- CBC, U&Es, LFTs,
- chest radiograph,
- peripheral blood cultures and blood cultures from all lumina of the central line if present (identify blood cultures taken from lines clearly),
- observations,
- take urine specimens and throat swabs for routine and viral cultures,
- if the patient has diarrhea, send a stool specimen, and
- if there is a focus of infection, a specimen should be taken from the appropriate site.

Neutropenic patients can be divided into three clinical groups:

1. Immunocompetent patients who present with neutropenia are compromised and require urgent treatment.
2. Immunocompromised patients who present with neutropenia are compromised and require urgent treatment.
3. Otherwise well patients with neutropenia: these patients may be known to be neutropenic previously or presenting anew and require investigation to look for an underlying diagnosis.

General Management

Any patient in whom there is a reasonable suspicion of neutropenia (i.e., chemotherapy within the previous 4 weeks) and demonstrate fever or a good history of fever detected by the patient before admission should be treated with broad-spectrum antibiotics. Most cancer treatment centers recommend delivering intravenous antibiotics within 1 h of presentation with possible neutropenic sepsis, and will advise patients to speak to, or attend, the treatment center directly rather than going to their GP.

Pharmacological Management

Empiric antibiotic treatment should be initiated immediately according to local policy. Granulocyte colony-stimulating factor (G-CSF) in neutropenia is a growth factor that is given subcutaneously and can stimulate the bone marrow, thus leading to an increased number of white cells. In some cases it is used prophylactically. G-CSF shortens the time taken for the neutrophil count to recover and treatment is usually reserved for neutropenia associated with severe or recurrent infections [20].

Opioid Overdose

Opioid overdose is rarely a problem in the palliative care setting, provided that the drugs are systematically titrated according to the pain assessment and reassessment. If the patient inadvertently takes more medication than advised then the subsequent dose can often be omitted and the patient observed. However, if the excessive opioid dose causes respiratory depression or coma, inpatient treatment is advised.

The specific antidote naloxone is indicated if there is coma or respiratory depression. As naloxone has a shorter duration of action than many opioids, close monitoring and repeated injections are necessary according to the respiratory rate and depth of coma. The dose requires careful titration to ensure that pain does not return.

When repeated administration of naloxone is required, it can be given by continuous intravenous infusion instead, and the rate of infusion adjusted according to vital signs [3]. The effects of some opioids, such as buprenorphine, are only partially reversed by naloxone. Dextropropoxyphene and methadone both have a very long duration of action and patients may need to be monitored for long periods following large overdoses.

Naloxone Dose

Opioid overdose can be treated with naloxone in the following ways:

- Intravenous injection, 0.4–2.0 mg. If there is no response, repeat at intervals of 2–3 min to a maximum of 10 mg (then review diagnosis). Further doses may be required if respiratory function deteriorates.
- Subcutaneous or intramuscular injection, the adult and child doses are the same as for intravenous injection. This route should only be used if the intravenous route is not feasible (because the onset of action is slower).
- Continuous intravenous infusion using an infusion pump, 4 mg diluted in 20 mL intravenous infusion solution (unlicensed concentration) at a rate adjusted according to response. The initial rate may be set at 60% of initial intravenous injection dose (see above) and infused over 1 h.

Seizures
Definition

A seizure is uncontrolled electrical activity in the brain, which may produce a physical convulsion, minor physical signs, thought disturbances, or a combination of symptoms.

Prevalence

Seizures (generalized or partial) occur in 10–15% of palliative care patients, most often due to primary or secondary brain tumors where it occurs in 20–35% of patients (Figure 5.8), cerebrovascular disease, epilepsy, or biochemical abnormalities (e.g., low sodium, hypercalcemia, uremia) [22].

Assessment

Exclude other causes of loss of consciousness or abnormal limb/facial movement (e.g., vasovagal episode, postural hypotension, arrhythmia, hypoglycemia, extrapyramidal adverse effects from dopamine antagonists, alcohol).

Determine whether the patient has had previous seizures or is at risk (history of epilepsy, previous secondary seizure, known cerebral disease). Is there a problem with usual antiepileptic drug therapy, is the patient unable to take oral medication, or are there drug interactions (e.g., corticosteroids reduce the effect of carbamazepine and phenytoin) [22]?

General Management

The following guidelines are for the general management of seizures:

- try to ensure that the patient does not fall or bump into any sharp objects,
- do not attempt to restrain the patient,
- do not try to force anything into the patient's mouth,

Risk of seizures according to tumor type	
Tumor type	Risk of seizures (%)
Dysembryoplastic neuroepithelial tumor, ganglioglioma	80–100
Low-grade astrocytoma	75
Meningioma	30–60
High-grade astrocytoma	30–50
Brain metastases	20–35
Primary CNS lymphoma	10

Figure 5.8 Risk of seizures according to tumor type. *CNS* central nervous system. (Data from Rossetti and Stupp [21])

- when the seizure stops, turn the patient on to the side,
- the patient will be sleepy for a while after the seizure,
- if the seizure does not stop by itself in about 5–10 min or if another seizure occurs soon after the first, call for medical assistance, and
- do not shout or expect verbal commands to be obeyed.

Seizures are frightening to the patient and family. Take time afterwards to explore the concerns of the patient and family and offer honest reassurance. Address questions such as whether the patient will swallow his or her tongue, or choke to death during a seizure, or whether there will be permanent brain damage.

Pharmacological Management

The response to pharmacological therapy is individualized and highly variable. The dose should be titrated to clinical response rather than to a specific serum level [4].

Acute Seizures

The following are options for the pharmacological management of acute seizures [22]:

- in hospital, iv diazepam in 2-mg bolus doses up to 10 mg, or lorazepam 4 mg by slow iv injection, are used,
- give diazepam rectal solution 10–30 mg pr or via a stoma,
- give midazolam 5 mg sc, repeated after 5 min,
- buccal midazolam 10 mg can be given using the parenteral preparation or the buccal liquid.

Persistent Seizures

The following are options for the pharmacological management of persistent seizures:

- intravenous phenytoin is used in hospital settings,
- phenobarbital can be given as 100 mg im bolus dose followed, if needed, by CSCI of phenobarbital 200–400 mg diluted in water for infusion over 24 h.

Chronic Seizure Control

Most patients with a structural cause for seizures benefit from treatment.

Partial or Secondary Qeneralized Seizures

The following are options for the pharmacological management of partial or secondary seizures:

- Sodium valproate should be given initially at 600 mg/day in two divided doses, preferably after food. This can be increased by 200 mg/day every 3 days to a maximum of 2.5 g/day. The usual maintenance dose is 1–2 g/day.

- Carbamazepine: for epilepsy, initially, 100–200 mg od/bd, increased slowly to a usual dose of 0.8–1.2 g/day in divided doses. In some cases 1.6–2 g/day in divided doses may be needed. In elderly patients, reduce the initial dose.

- Lamotrigine: for the monotherapy of seizures initially 25 mg od for 14 days, increased to 50 mg od for further 14 days, then increased by maximum of 100 mg every 7–14 days. The usual maintenance is 100–200 mg/day in one to two divided doses. For the adjunctive therapy of seizures with valproate, initially 25 mg on alternate days for 14 days, then 25 mg od for a further 14 days, thereafter increased by maximum of 50 mg every 7–14 days. The usual maintenance is 100–200 mg/day in one to two divided doses. For adjunctive therapy of seizures (with enzyme-inducing drugs) without valproate, initially 50 mg od for 14 days, then 50 mg bd for further 14 days, thereafter increased by maximum of 100 mg every 7–14 days. The usual maintenance is 200–400 mg/day in two divided doses.

Primary Generalized Seizures

The following are options for the pharmacological management of primary generalized seizures:

- sodium valproate: as above,
- lamotrigine: as above.

Dying Patient Unable to Take Oral Medication

The following are options for the pharmacological management of patients unable to take oral medication:

- anticonvulsants have a long half-life, so additional treatment may not be needed,
- midazolam 5 mg sc or diazepam rectal solution 10 mg pr, if required,
- midazolam 20–30 mg CSCI/24 h can be used as maintenance therapy.

If a seizure has occurred and recurrence is likely, then treatment is warranted [23]:

- The use of prophylactic anticonvulsant therapy in patients with brain tumors or metastases is controversial. It has not been shown to provide an advantage in seizure control.
- Seizure prophylaxis should be instituted after the first seizure.
- Clonazepam can be used for the temporary treatment of seizures not controlled by ongoing therapy.
- Start with clonazepam 0.5 mg po tds and then increase by 0.5 mg every 3 days until symptoms are controlled. As abrupt withdrawal of clonazepam after long-term use may precipitate status epilepticus, taper the dosage instead.
- Although diazepam has been the benzodiazepine of choice for status epilepticus, recent evidence indicates that lorazepam may be more beneficial because it provides longer control of seizures and produces less cardiorespiratory depression.
- Gabapentin can be used for adjuvant therapy of partial seizure and tonic–clonic seizures. The starting dose is 300 mg po tds/qds with a maintenance dose of 900–3,600 mg/day.
- Midazolam can be given intravenously, subcutaneously, or orally, with the quickest onset of action by the intravenous route. The intramuscular route is not recommended. Use a lower dose in older adults (1–2 mg).
- Phenobarbital is effective in both partial and generalized tonic–clonic seizures.

- Phenothiazines should be avoided in patients in whom cerebral irritation is a potential problem.
- Consider starting or increasing dexamethasone po or sc in seizures due to a brain tumor or metastasis. Dexamethasone should not be the only drug used, even if only one seizure has occurred.

Superior Vena Cava Obstruction
Definition
Superior vena cava obstruction (SVCO) or superior vena cava syndrome (SVCS) results from the direct obstruction of the SVC by malignancies.

Prevalence
SVCO occurs in 3–8% of patients with lung cancer (small- and squamous cell types) and lymphoma, and less frequently in breast and testicular cancer. It is found most commonly with right-sided lung tumors presenting with right-sided symptoms (up to 10% will develop SVCO) and occurs most frequently in cancer of the lung (70% of cases) or lymphoma (8%) [23].

Assessment
SVCO is due to compression, obstruction, or thrombosis impairing venous return (Figure 5.9) [24]. If active intervention is appropriate, admission will be required for assessment and possible chemotherapy, radiotherapy, or stenting.

Symptoms
The symptoms of SVCO are as follows [24]:
- dyspnea,
- facial/upper body and arms swelling and/or skin mottling (Figure 5.10) [25],
- headaches or 'muzziness',
- cough, and
- dysphagia.

Causes of superior vena cava obstruction	
Malignant causes	Lung carcinoma • Small-cell histology • Non-small-cell histology Lymphoma • Hodgkin's disease • Non-Hodgkin's lymphoma Metastatic carcinoma: many primary sites reported Esophageal carcinoma or leiomyoma Thyroid carcinoma Thymoma and thymic carcinoma Germ-cell tumouts Breast carcinoma Mesothelioma Leukemia: acute myeloid
Benign causes	Cardiac • Aneurysm of aorta or large arteries • Arteriovenous fistula • Congenital cardiac defects + surgical repair • Constrictive pericarditis Mediastinal fibrosis Sarcoidosis Pulmonary • Mediastinal emphysema • Tension pneumothorax Trauma Infection Arteritis Retrosternal goiter Thrombosis
Related to central venous lines	Pacemakers Parenteral feeding lines 'Hickman' lines Dialysis lines Swan–Ganz catheters 'Emergency' central lines LeVeen shunts

Figure 5.9 Causes of superior vena cava obstruction. (Data from Ostler et al. [24])

Signs

The signs of SVCO are as follows:

- swelling of the face and neck, and
- prominent blood vessels in the neck, trunk, and arms.

Superior vena cava obstruction

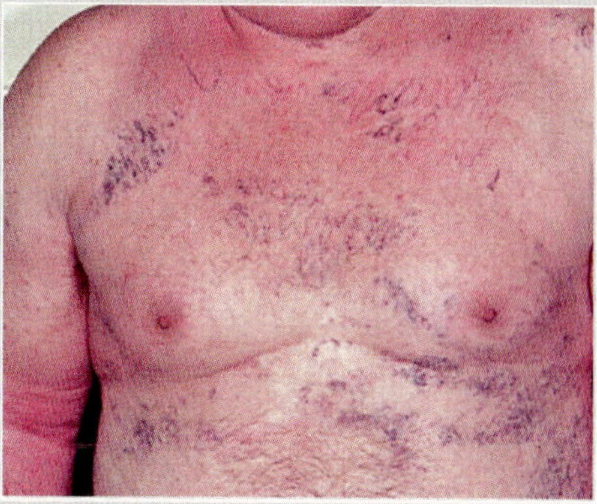

Figure 5.10 Superior vena cava obstruction. (Reproduced with permission from Elsevier [25])

Investigations

Investigations for SVCO are:

- chest CT scan, and
- chest radiograph and obtain histology via bronchoscopy, mediastinoscopy, or other accessible site.

After treatment, the average survival is 8 months. If the patient is bed-bound, terminal, refusing treatment, or after discussion with oncologist no further treatment is available, all symptom control and care measures should be given, and nursing support arranged (seek specialist advice).

Management

Immediately start dexamethasone (16 mg/day), which reduces the edema associated with the mediastinal tumor and helps prevent radio-therapy-induced inflammation.

There are three important treatments options [26]:

1. Vascular stenting may be considered. The insertion of a self-expanding metal stent into the SVC is a relatively new form of treatment. Thrombolysis may need to be performed before stent insertion, but the immediate and long-term effects are good, with

over 90% of patients dying without recurrence of SVCO. It is useful for rapid-onset SVCO and where histology is awaited.

2. Chemotherapy may be the treatment of choice in lymphoma and small-cell lung carcinoma (if diagnosis previously established).

3. Radiotherapy may be the treatment of choice if a mediastinal tumor is the cause.

In cases of recurrent SVCO:

- retrial of dexamethasone,
- radiotherapy may be considered, and
- vascular stent may be replaced.

Supportive Palliative Care

These interventions may be required alongside definitive treatments or if definitive treatment has failed:

- oxygen/heliox,
- low-dose opioids,
- benzodiazepines, and
- anxiety relaxation techniques.

References

1. Falk S, Reid C. Emergencies. In: Fallon M, Hanks G, editors. ABC of palliative care. 2nd ed. Oxford: Blackwell Publishing; 2006. p. 40–3.
2. Harris DG, Noble SI. Management of terminal hemorrhage in patients with advanced cancer: a systematic literature review. J Pain Symptom Manage. 2009;38:913–27.
3. British National Formulary. BNF 61. London: BMJ Group and Pharmaceutical Press; 2011. Available at: www.bnf.org. Last accessed 27 Nov 2011.
4. Palliative Drugs. Essential independent drug information for palliative and hospice care. Formulary 2011. Available at: www.palliativedrugs.com. Last accessed 27 Nov 2011.
5. Pereira J, Phan T. Management of bleeding in patients with advanced cancer. Oncologist. 2004;9:561–70.
6. Green D, Thompson JA, Montgomery B. Oncologic emergencies. In: Irwin RS, Rippe JM, editors. Intensive care medicine. 6th ed. Philadelphia: Lippincott Williams & Wilkins; 2008. p. 1419–30.
7. Bower M, Cox S. Endocrine and metabolic complications of advanced cancer. In: Hanks G, Cherny N, Kaasa S, et al., editors. Oxford textbook of palliative medicine. 4th ed. Oxford: Oxford University Press; 2010. p. 1015–33.
8. Clines GA, Guise TA. Hypercalcaemia of malignancy and basic research on mechanisms responsible for osteolytic and osteoblastic metastasis to bone. Endocr Relat Cancer. 2005;12:549–83.

9.   Ralston SH, Coleman R, Fraser WD, et al. Cancer-associated hypercalcemia: morbidity and mortality. Clinical experience in 126 treated patients. Ann Intern Med. 1990;112:499–504.

10. Hemphill RR. Hypercalcemia. Available at: www.emedicine.medscape.com/article/240681-overview. Last accessed 27 Nov 2011.

11. Waters M. Hypercalcaemia. InnovAiT. 2009;2:698–701.

12. Loblaw DA, Perry J, Chambers A, et al. A population-based study of malignant spinal cord compression in Ontario. Clin Oncol. 2003;15:211–7.

13. Bach F, Larsen BH, Rohde K, et al. Metastatic spinal cord compression. Occurrence, symptoms, clinical presentations, and prognosis in 398 patients with spinal cord compression. Acta Neurochir. 1990;107:37–43.

14. Conway R, Graham J, Kidd J, Levack P. What happens to people after malignant cord compression? Survival, function, quality of life, emotional well-being and place of care 1 month after diagnosis. Clin Oncol. 2007;19:56–62.

15. Akram H, Allibone J. Spinal surgery for palliation in malignant spinal cord compression. Clin Oncol. 2010;22:792–800.

16. National Institute for Health and Clinical Excellence. Metastatic spinal cord compression. NICE clinical guidelines 75. London: National Collaborating Centre for Cancer; 2008.

17. George R, Jeba J, Ramkumar G, et al. Interventions for the treatment of metastatic extradural spinal cord compression in adults. Cochrane Database Syst Rev. 2008;(4):CD006716.

18. Eleraky M, Papanastassiou I, Vrionis FD. Management of metastatic spine disease. Curr Opin Support Palliat Care. 2010;4:182–8.

19. National Institute for Health and Clinical Excellence. Neutropenic sepsis: prevention and management of neutropenic sepsis in cancer patients. Scope. Available at: www.nice.org.uk/nicemedia/live/12349/49068/49068.pdf. Last accessed 27 Nov 2011.

20. Oppenheim BA, Anderson H. Management of febrile neutropenia in low risk cancer patients. Thorax. 2000;55 suppl 1:S63–9.

21. Rossetti AO, Stupp R. Epilepsy in brain tumor patients. Curr Opin Neurol. 2010;23:603–9.

22. Palliative Care Guidelines. Emergencies in palliative care. Available at: www.palliativecareguidelines.scot.nhs.uk/documents/Seizures.pdf. Last accessed 27 Nov 2011.

23. Fraser Health. Hospice palliative care program symptom guidelines: twitching/myoclonus/seizures. 2006. Available at: www.fraserhealth.ca/media/19FHSymptomGuidelinesMyoclonus.pdf. Last accessed 27 Nov 2011.

24. Ostler PJ, Clarke DP, Watkinson AF, Gaze MN. Superior vena cava obstruction: a modern management strategy. Clin Oncol. 1997;9:83–9.

25. Falk S, Fallon M. ABC of palliative care: emergencies. 1997. Available at: www.bmj.com/content/315/7121/1525.full. Last accessed 27 Nov 2011.

26. Rowell NP, Gleeson FV. Steroids, radiotherapy, chemotherapy and stents for superior vena caval obstruction in carcinoma of the bronchus. Cochrane Database Syst Rev. 2001;(4):CD001316.

Chapter 6

Advance Care Planning

ACP is a voluntary process of discussion about future care between individuals and their care providers, irrespective of discipline. If individuals wish, their family and friends may be included. It is recommended that with individuals' agreement this discussion is documented, regularly reviewed, and communicated to the key people involved in their care [1].

An ACP discussion might include the following [1]:

- individuals' concerns and wishes,
- their important values or personal goals for care,
- their understanding about their illness and prognosis, and
- their preferences and wishes for types of care or treatment that may be beneficial in the future and the availability of these.

ACP involves a number of processes:

- informing the patient,
- eliciting preferences,
- identifying a surrogate decision-maker to act if patients no longer able to make decisions about their own care, and
- discussions with family members, or at least with the person who is to be the surrogate decision-maker.

The principle of ACP is not new. It is common for patients aware of approaching death to discuss with their carers how they wish to be treated; however, these wishes have not always been respected, especially

G. Zeppetella, *Palliative Care in Clinical Practice*,
DOI 10.1007/978-1-4471-2843-4_6,
© Springer-Verlag London 2012

Principles of a good death

- To know when death is coming and to understand what can be expected
- To be able to retain control of what happens
- To be afforded dignity and privacy
- To have control over pain relief and other symptom control
- To have choice and control over where death occurs (at home or elsewhere)
- To have access to information and expertise of whatever kind is necessary
- To have access to any spiritual or emotional support required
- To have access to hospice care in any location, not only in hospital
- To have control over who is present and who shares the end
- To be able to issue advance directives which ensure that wishes are respected
- To have time to say goodbye, and control over other aspects of timing
- To be able to leave when it is time to go, and not to have life prolonged pointlessly

Figure 6.1 Principles of a good death. (Data from Smith [2]. Reproduced with permission from BMJ Publishing Group)

if the patient is urgently taken to hospital and there is disagreement among family members about what is appropriate treatment. To help prevent this, a number of processes, as part of the end-of-life care pathway, can be used to help facilitate and empower patient wishes (Fig. 6.1) [2].

Stages of Death and Dying

A number of stages in death and dying have been identified as follows (Fig. 6.2) [1, 3, 4]:

- Shock and denial: the patient's initial reaction is shock, followed by denial that anything is wrong. Some patients never pass beyond this stage and may go doctor shopping until they find one who supports their position.
- Anger: at this stage, patients become frustrated, irritable, and angry that they are ill, asking, "Why me?" Patients in this stage are difficult to manage because their anger is displaced on to doctors, hospital staff, church/God, and family. Sometimes the anger is directed at themselves in the belief that illness has occurred as a punishment for wrongdoing.
- Bargaining: the patient may attempt to negotiate with physicians, friends, or even God, that, in return for a cure, he or she will fulfill

Key principles of the advance care planning process

- The process is voluntary. No pressure should be brought to bear by the professional, the family, or any organization on the individual concerned to take part in ACP

- ACP must be a patient-centered dialogue over a period of time

- The process of ACP is a reflection of society's desire to respect personal autonomy. The content of any discussion should be determined by the individual concerned. The individual may not wish to confront future issues; this should be respected

- All health- and social care staff should be open to any discussion which may be instigated by an individual and know how to respond to their questions

- Health- and social care staff should instigate ACP only if in the context of a professional judgment that leads them to believe that it is likely to benefit the care of the individual. The discussion should be introduced sensitively

- Staff will require the appropriate training to enable them to communicate effectively and to understand the legal and ethical issues involved

- Staff need to be aware when they have reached the limits of their knowledge and competence and know when and from whom to seek advice

- Discussion should focus on the views of individuals, although they may wish to invite their carer or another close family member or friend to participate. Some families may have discussed their issues and would welcome an approach to share this discussion

- Confidentiality should be respected in line with current good practice and professional guidance

- Health- and social care staff should be aware, and give a realistic account, of the support, services, and choices available in the particular circumstances. This should entail referral to an appropriate colleague or agency when necessary

- The professional must have adequate knowledge of the benefits, harms, and risks associated with treatment to enable the individual to make an informed decision

- Choice in terms of place of care will influence treatment options, because certain treatments may not be available at home or in a care home, eg, chemotherapy or intravenous therapy. Individuals may need to be admitted to hospital for symptom management, or to a hospice or hospital because support is not available at home

- ACP requires that the individual has the capacity to understand, discuss options available, and agree to what is then planned. Agreement should be documented

- Should an individual wish to make a decision to refuse treatment (advance decision) they should be guided by a professional with appropriate knowledge and this should be documented according to the requirements of the Mental Capacity Act 2005

Figure 6.2 Key principles of the advance care planning process. *ACP* advance care planning (Data from UK National Health Service End of Life Care Programme [1])

one or many promises, e.g., give to charity or attend church regularly.

- Depression: the patient shows clinical signs of depression (e.g., withdrawal, hopelessness, psychomotor retardation, sleep disturbances, and possibly suicidal thoughts). The depression may be a reaction to the effects of the illness on his or her life (e.g., loss of job, economic hardship, isolation from friends and family) or it may be in anticipation of the actual loss of life that will occur shortly.

- Acceptance: the person realizes that death is inevitable and accepts its universality.

Home Care of the Dying Patient

Given the option, most people would prefer to die at home surrounded by their loved ones. However, carers may require support and resources to help them to cope [4]. This can mean that a close person such as a spouse, long-term partner, or close relative is available 24 h a day. The caregiver must be prepared to cope with both the emotional and physical needs of the patient, which can be very demanding if the patient is to have a 'good' death (Fig. 6.1) [2].

There can also be a significant burden upon the community-based services in terms of time and emotion. Care of the dying patient at home requires a team approach involving the GP or family practitioner, district nurses, perhaps Macmillan nurses, and any other professionals with input such as Social Services (see Fig. 1.2). If there is likely to be any problem out-of-hours, the local provider of out-of-hours care should be informed. A holistic assessment is required so that all areas of care are covered (Fig. 6.3) [5].

Fear is common, as are questions about the prognosis or the manner of the deterioration. It is important to answer questions to the best of one's ability, being honest about the certainties and uncertainties. Most patients are not seeking straight answers, and as the relationship with them develops it will be easier to know how much they want to know, when they want to know it, and how they want to hear it.

People in the final stages of their illness generally become weaker and spend a greater proportion of their time in bed. They also become drowsier and less able to take fluids or food, or swallow medication. It may then be necessary to consider a more appropriate approach to caring and nursing, e.g., by discontinuing medications that are no longer required or by using alternative routes of administration for those still needed. In essence all nursing care will now focus on ensuring comfort, safety, and support. The physical changes too, such as urinary or fecal incontinence,

Areas that require assessment

- Current symptoms
- Patient emotional state
- Patient spiritual state
- Medication regimen
- Physical examination
- Patient understanding of the extent of the disease, options for treatment, and prognosis
- Patient wishes with respect to medical information and participation in decision-making
- Patient wishes with respect to information release to significant others and wishes with respect to medical information and participation in decision-making
- Patient wishes with respect to care setting; lay caregiver wishes with respect to care setting
- Patient goals
- Current formal home care support services
- Lay caregiver education, physical and emotional support needs
- Home physical arrangements
- Clarify existence/absence of an advance statement or decision
- Resuscitation status
- Patient financial needs

Figure 6.3 Areas that require assessment. (Data from Taube [5])

are distressing for the patient, unpleasant for the caregiver, and add to the burden of caring.

Caring for a loved one who is dying is a demanding time. The emotional turmoil, compounded perhaps by a lack of sleep, must take its toll. Seeing one's parent, sibling, or spouse/partner slipping from a strong and independent person to a frail, dependent, incontinent, and perhaps at times confused shadow of his or her former self is most distressing and can produce feelings of anger or guilt.

Caregivers, similar to the patient, need to know what to expect. They may find the 'death rattle' of terminal breathing or Cheyne–Stokes breathing most distressing. Practical details should not be forgotten, such as who to call in case of need and what to do when death occurs, including that it is not necessary to call the paramedics.

The following sections provide information on the tools and processes available to assess, monitor, plan ahead, and support patients, caregivers, and healthcare professionals.

Gold Standards Framework

The GSF is a systematic evidence-based approach to optimizing the care for patients nearing the end of life delivered by generalist providers. It is concerned with helping people to live well until the end of life and includes care in the final years of life for people with any end-stage illness in any setting (see www.goldstandardsframework.nhs.uk). The GSF is intended to be a generic improvement tool and, although developed for primary care by primary care, initially for cancer patients, it can be used for any patient with a life-limiting illness and in other settings such as care homes.

The following are the five goals of the GSF [6]:

1. consistent high-quality care,
2. alignment with patients' preferences,
3. pre-planning and anticipation of needs,
4. improved staff confidence and teamwork, and
5. more home-based, less hospital-based care.

The GSF embodies an approach that centers on the needs of patients and their families, and encourages interprofessional primary care teams to work together. The GSF is underpinned by the best available evidence of key issues and effective solutions in this field, and at every stage there has been concurrent evaluation and research. Primary care teams find that it affirms their good practice, standardizes quality palliative care activities, and improves consistency of care. Practice review and audit are an integral part of the GSF, as are measures to improve consistency and dependability of care provided.

In 2009, the Royal College of General Practitioners in the UK approved the College's End of life Care Strategy, supporting further progress with GSF. In June 2009, the fully refreshed and revised GSF Primary Care Next Stage Programme 'Going for Gold' was launched with a new training program, support, and resources to support practice teams to move on to the next stage with use of GSF in their teams (Fig. 6.4) [6].

Three triggers for palliative care are suggested to identify those patients for whom we can use any combination of the following methods:

**The Gold Standards Framework for palliative care in primary healthcare
The seven Cs:**

Communication	Practices have a register of patients near the end of life that allows teams to prioritize care. The Prognostic Indicator Guidance, including the 'surprise question,' is one of the tools to identify patients for the register
Coordination	Record key contacts, eg, usual district nurse(s) and GPs (not just the senior partner) and their contact information. Liaise closely about changes and discharges. GP reception staff are highly trained, often aware of the GSF patients and GP movements and so can be auseful link
Control of symptoms	Ensure that there is easy access locally to specialist palliative care advice for GPs, nurses, community matrons, care homes, out-of-hours clinicians, ambulance staff, and pharmacists
Continuity	Passport information describes accessible brief patient details, which enable the patient and family to access good care wherever they are, eg, in the emergency department with no other notes
	Have clear systems in place for liaison with other professionals, eg, out-of-hours services, pharmacists, hospital and specialist nurses, and ambulance staff
Continued learning	The GSF encourages reflection on individual cases to improve systems of care. Identify local needs across primary care and offer appropriate solutions
Carer support	Ensure that carers are supported on discharge for a smooth transition and seamless care.ensure that carers have the opportunity to discuss or read about what may happen at the end of life and how to deal with this
Care of the dying	Ensure that the systematic approach taken, such as I theriverpool Care Pathway or GSF minimum protocol, is transferable to all settings. Offer the patient realistic choices of place of care, document, and act on their preferences

Figure 6.4 The Gold Standards Framework for palliative care in primary healthcare: The seven Cs. (Data from Thomas [6])

1. Would you be surprised if this patient were to die in the next 6–12 months? If not, what measures might be taken to improve quality of life now and in preparation for the dying stage?
2. Choice/need: the patient with advanced disease makes a choice for comfort care only, not 'curative' treatment, or is in special need of supportive/palliative care, e.g., refusing renal transplantation.
3. Clinical indicators: specific indicators of advanced disease for each of the three main end-of-life patient groups – cancer, organ failure, elderly frail/dementia.

The GSF Toolkit comprises a number of templates and tools that enable delivery of GSF in various settings. For further information visit www. goldstandardsframework.nhs.uk.

Preferred Priorities of Care

Although people's preferences and priorities may change as death approaches, these changes will be linked on occasion to concerns about the availability of services for their preferred place of care. The main findings can be summarized as follows:

- Most people would prefer to be cared for at home, as long as high-quality care can be assured and as long as they do not place too great a burden on their families and carers.
- Some research has shown that some people (particularly older people) who live alone wish to live at home for as long as possible, although they wish to die elsewhere where they can be certain not to be on their own.
- Some people, on the other hand, would not wish to be cared for at home, because they do not want family members to have to care for them. Many of these people would prefer to be cared for in a hospice.
- Most, but not all, people would prefer not to die in a hospital – although this is in fact where most people do die.

The PPC is a patient-held document designed to facilitate patient choice in relation to end-of-life issues by recording what their wishes and preferences are during the last year or months of life [7]. The document was originally developed for people who had cancer and living at home, and focused on where they wanted to be cared for when they were dying. Recently it has been expanded to include other wishes and preferences that people might have when they are coming toward the end of their life.

The PPC document (Fig. 6.5) provides the opportunity to discuss difficult issues that may not otherwise be addressed, to the detriment of patient care. The explicit recording of patients'/carers' wishes can form the basis of care planning in multidisciplinary teams and other services, minimizing inappropriate admissions and interventions. Individuals can

Discussing the Preferred Priorities for Care document

- How you feel about your disease, what you understand about your illness, and what your outlook is

- Fears that you may have such as being in pain, or being a burden to your family

- Particular needs that those caring for you may have

- Who you would like to care for you now and in the future

- Where you would like to die – at home, or in a hospice or hospital

- What you do and don't want to be told, eg, how long you have to live

- Anything you'd like to do while there is still time

Figure 6.5 Discussing the preferred priorities for care document. (Data from UK National Health Service End of Life Care Programme [7])

initiate the PPC at any time and this will help staff follow their wishes in making best-interest decisions if the individual loses capacity toward the end of life.

Patients with cancer are more likely to receive end-of-life care that is consistent with their preferences when they have had the opportunity to discuss their wishes [8]. The PPC is not a legal document but is covered by the Mental Capacity Act 2005. If the patient becomes unable to make a decision about his or her care, the document has to be taken into account. For further information visit: www.endoflifecareforadults.nhs.uk.

Liverpool Care Pathway

The LCP is an integrated care pathway that is used at the bedside to improve the quality of the dying in the last hours and days of life. Integrated pathways describe the patient's journey and help ensure that he or she receives appropriate care throughout (Fig. 6.6) [9]. They aim to predict possible problems that the person may have, and hopefully prevent them.

The idea behind the LCP is to care for people who are dying in the same way, wherever they are. It covers all aspects of care including the following [9]:

- keeping patients comfortable by controlling their symptoms,

- when to prescribe certain drugs to prevent symptoms before they start,

- when to discontinue some treatments or aspects of care,

Integrated care pathways

- Focused on the patient and his or her family
- Based on evidence
- Involve the patient and his or her carers
- Set standards for how things should be done
- Involve all professionals caring for the patient and his or her family

Figure 6.6 Integrated care pathways. (Data from Ellershaw and Wilkinson [9])

Key Liverpool Care Pathway messages

1. The LCP is only as good as the people using it
2. The LCP should not be used without the support of education and training
3. Good communication is pivotal to success
4. The LCP neither hastens nor postpones death
5. Diagnosis of dying should be made by the multidisciplinary team
6. The LCP does not recommend the use of continuous deep sedation
7. The LCP does not preclude the use of artificial hydration
8. The LCP support continual reassessment
9. Reflect, audit, measure, and learn
10. Stop, think, assess, and change

Figure 6.7 Key Liverpool Care Pathway messages. *LCP* Liverpool Care Pathway (Data from Ellershaw and Wilkinson [9])

- psychological and spiritual support, and
- support for the family.

The LCP aims to transfer the best quality for care of the dying from the hospice movement into other clinical areas, so that wherever the person is dying there can be an equitable model of care. The LCP (Fig. 6.7) [9] has been implemented in hospitals, care homes, the individual's own home/community, and hospices. The LCP is not the answer to all our needs for care of the dying but it is a step in the right direction. It is recommended as a best practice model, most recently, by the Department of Health in the UK [10].

The LCP is a process divided into five sections:

1. assessment,
2. clinical decision,

3. communication,
4. management, and
5. reassessment.

The LCP aims to support and not replace clinical judgment. It enables healthcare professionals to focus on care in the last hours or days of life and provide high-quality care tailored to the patient's individual needs when death is expected, e.g., the LCP does not preclude the use of clinically assisted nutrition, hydration, or antibiotics. All clinical decisions must be made in the patient's best interest.

The recognition and diagnosis of dying are always complex, and uncertainty is an integral part of dying. There are occasions when a patient who is thought to be dying lives longer than expected, and vice versa. Seek a second opinion or specialist palliative care support as needed. Changes in care at this complex, uncertain time are made in the best interest of the patient and relative or carer, and need to be reviewed regularly by the multidisciplinary team (Fig. 6.8) [11].

Common symptoms at the end of life include:

- pain,
- nausea,
- agitation,
- respiratory secretions, and
- dyspnea.

For LCP symptom algorithms see Figs. 8.12, 8.13, 8.14, 8.15, and 8.16.

Death at Home

At present most deaths in England occur in NHS hospitals (58%), with deaths at home (18%) and in care homes (17%) collectively accounting for approximately 35% of all deaths [12]. Hospices account for approximately 4% of deaths, with approximately 3% occurring in other locations [13].

Many patients wish to die at home provided that high-quality care can be assured and that they and their families feel well supported. The mode of death of many terminally ill patients can be anticipated. An explanation of progressive loss of consciousness and awareness, and how

Decision-making in the Liverpool Care Pathway

Decision-making in: diagnosing, dying, and use of the LCP supporting care in the final hours or days of life

Assessment

Deterioration in the patient's condition suggests that the patient could be dying

Multidisciplinary team (MDT) assessment

- Is there a potentially reversible cause for the patient's condition, eg, exclude opioid toxicity, renal failure, hypercalcemia, infection
- Could the patient be in the last hours or days of life?
- Is specialist referral needed? eg, specialist palliative care or a second opinion

Clinical decision

Patient is NOT diagnosed as dying (in the last hours or days of life)

Patient is diagnosed as dying (in the last hours or days of life)

Review the current plan of care

Patient, relative, or carer communication is focused on recognition and understanding that the patient is dying

Communication

Discussion with the patient and relative or carer to explain the new or revised plan of care

Discussion with the patient, relative, or carer (IMCA as required) to explain the current plan of care and use of the LCP

The LCP for the Dying Patient is commenced, including ongoing regular assessments

Management

Reassessment

A full MDT reassessment and review of the current plan of care should be triggered when 1 or more of the following apply:

Improved conscious level, functional ability, oral intake, mobility, ability to perform self-care

and/ or

Concerns expressed regarding management plan from either patient, relative, carer, or team member

and/ or

It is 3 days since the last full MDT assessment

Figure 6.8 Decision-making in the Liverpool Care Pathway. *LCP* Liverpool Care Pathway, *IMCA* Independent Mental Capacity Advocate (Reproduced with kind permission from the LCP Central Team at the Marie Curie Palliative Care Institute Liverpool [11])

symptoms can be managed, will help lessen anxiety. Careful implementation of tools such as the LCP will help ensure that the patient is regularly reviewed, symptoms are adequately managed, and families know what to expect and what they should do once death occurs [9].

Do-not-attempt resuscitation (DNAR) decisions are an important element of care, and once made need to be communicated effectively. Since 2001, hospital trusts have been required to have resuscitation policies in place to support people's choices about care; the situation in the community is less consistent. One way of ensuring that futile attempts to resuscitate are not attempted is to encourage the family not to telephone the emergency services, because without previous information paramedics may feel duty bound to attempt resuscitation on arrival.

After the patient's death the relatives usually contact the GP or family practitioner; outside normal office hours this may be a doctor who does not know the patient or the circumstances of the death. In advising patients of the requirements after death, it is usually sufficient to explain the need for certification and registration of the death, and to assure them that when they contact a funeral undertaker they will get all the necessary support and advice. Written information for bereaved relatives is available from the Department of Social Security [14, 15]. Relatives may ask, at this time, for equipment or medication to be removed. Although the syringe driver can be easily detached and the battery removed, other equipment is usually removed at a later date, often after contacting the district nursing team. Any prescribed medication is the patient's property and should not be removed by the clinician. The relatives can be advised to take the medication to their pharmacist where it can be properly destroyed.

A doctor who attended the patient during his or her last illness, commonly the GP or family practitioner, will usually issue a medical certificate of the cause of death. If the body is to be buried there is no legal requirement for it to be seen by a doctor after death, although it is advisable to do so. It is then the responsibility of the family to register the death at the register office. In England and Wales, families normally need to register the death within 5 days and usually at the register office in the area where the person died.

If it was the wish of the deceased to donate the organs for transplantation, or the whole body for medical teaching purposes, some haste is required to ensure that this can happen. The most common organ donated in a palliative care setting is the cornea which can be removed from the body up to 24 h after death. The usual procedure is to approach the next of kin to make sure that they do not object to organ donation.

If the body is to be cremated it must first be seen by the certifying doctor and by a second, independent medical practitioner whose registration is of at least 5 years' standing and who is not a partner or a relative of the first doctor or of the deceased. The Cremation Regulations 2008 came into effect on January 1 2009 and were intended to modernize and consolidate all previous regulations, replacing the Cremation Regulations 1930 [16].

There are instances when the death is reported to the coroner. These include where it appears that [17]:

- no doctor attended the deceased during his or her last illness,
- although a doctor attended during the last illness, thedeceased was not seen either within 14 days before death orafter death,
- the cause of death appears to be unknown,
- death occurred during an operation or before recovery from the effects of an anesthetic,
- the death was due to an industrial accident, disease, or poisoning,
- the death was sudden or unexpected,
- the death was unnatural,
- the death was due to violence or neglect,
- the death was in other suspicious circumstances, and
- the death occurred in prison or police custody.

In most cases there is no need to report the death to the coroner's officer. The most common reason in a palliative care setting is to discuss patients with an industrial-related disease such a mesothelioma. It should be noted that, if the doctor called to certify the death was not made aware beforehand that death was expected, the coroner may still be contacted because, as far as the attending doctor is concerned, the death was sudden or unexpected. Clearly this causes unnecessary distress to the family and could be avoided. Adopting a tool such as the GSF where continuity is a key element of the process can help minimize such problems.

Bereavement Care

Bereavement refers to the period of mourning and grief following the death of a beloved person or animal. The word bereavement comes from an ancient Germanic root word meaning 'to rob' or 'to seize by violence.'

Mourning is the overt expression of grief and the usual response to bereavement. Frequently it is culturally modified and influenced. Grief refers to the feelings of sorrow, anger, guilt, and confusion that arise when one experiences a loss. It is the effect or emotion that accompanies bereavement. Bereavement is a highly individual and complex experience that can give rise to a wide range of changes and needs, practical, financial, social, emotional, and spiritual (Fig. 6.9) [18].

Preparatory Grief

Preparatory grief is a normal reaction that people experience when they are preparing for death. The symptoms of preparatory grief can be very similar to those of depression, but management is different, so the two should be distinguished.

The following distinguished preparatory grief from depression:
• mood changes with time,
• normal self-esteem,

Normal grief: expected changes				
Physical	**Functional**	**Intrapersonal**	**Intrapersonal**	**Spiritual**
Sleeping patterns	Activities of daily living	Relationships Family roles	Mood Stress levels	Beliefs
Energy level	Economic status	Social status	Concentration	The search for understanding
Sexual function	Productivity at work or school	Social skills	Thoughts of dying, death, life, and living	The search for purpose and meaning
Blood pressure				
Digestive processes			Focus on health	The need to ask the 'big' questions
General health			Sense of self and identity	

Figure 6.9 **Normal grief: expected changes**. (Data from Egan and Arnold [18])

- enjoying seeing friends and family, and
- looking forward to special occasions.

Four stages or phases have been identified in uncomplicated bereavement (Fig. 6.10).

Common symptoms of grief include changes in appetite and weight, fatigue, insomnia and other sleep disturbances, loss of interest in sex, low energy levels, nausea and vomiting, chest or throat pain, and headache. People who have lost a loved one in traumatic circumstances may have such symptoms of post-traumatic stress disorder as an exaggerated startle response, visual or auditory hallucinations, or high levels of muscular tension.

Bereavement can be associated with an excess risk of mortality, a higher prevalence of physical and mental symptoms and illnesses, and an increased use of medical services [19]. Most people find a way of adjusting to the loss, but some may find it too difficult or traumatic without additional support. There are a number of situations, however, that can affect or prolong the grief process (Fig. 6.11) [20].

There are principally four tasks involved in mourning:

1. accept the reality of the loss,
2. work through the pain of grief,

Phases in uncomplicated bereavement	
Phase	**Notes**
Shock, disbelief, feelings of numbness	This initial phase lasts about 2 weeks, during which the bereaved person finally accepts the reality of the loved one's death
Suffering the pain of grief	This phase typically lasts for several months. Some people undergo a mild temporary depression approximately 6 months after the loved one's death
Adjusting to life without the loved one	In this phase of bereavement, survivors may find themselves taking on the loved one's roles and responsibilities as well as redefining their own identities
Moving forward with life	Most people reach this stage within 1–2 years after the loved one's death. Forming new relationships and having positive expectations of the future

Figure 6.10 Phases in uncomplicated bereavement

Prolonged grief

- An unexpected or violent death
- Suicide of a loved one
- Lack of a support system or friendships
- Traumatic childhood experiences, such as abuse or neglect
- Childhood separation anxiety
- Close ordependent relationship to the deceased person
- Being unprepared for the death
- In the case of a child's death, the number of remaining children
- Lack of resilience or adaptability to life changes

Figure 6.11 Prolonged grief. (Data from Worden [20])

Facilitating grief

- Help thesurvivor 'actualize' the loss
- Help thesurvivor to identify and express feelings
- Assist living without the deceased person
- Facilitate emotional withdrawal from the deceased person
- Provide time to grieve
- Interpret normal behavior
- Allow for individual differences
- Provide continuing support
- Examine defenses
- Identify pathology and refer

Figure 6.12 Facilitating grief. (Data from Worden [20])

3. adjust to an environment in which the deceased person is missing, and

4. emotionally relocate the deceased person and move on with life.

Helping people through grief can entail normalizing a number of processes (Fig. 6.12) [20]. Long-term support is sometimes required through bereavement counseling and peer support groups.

Many healthcare professionals may find the deaths of certain patients emotionally draining. It is important to find means of support. Colleagues or peers may be able to offer such support; if they cannot, other sources should be sought such as a mentor, a friend, or a community leader.

References

1. National Health Service End of Life Care Programme. Advance care planning: a guide for health and social care staff. 2008. Available at www.endoflifecareforadults.nhs.uk/assets/downloads/pubs_Advance_Care_Planning_guide.pdf. Last accessed 27 Nov 2011.

2. Smith R. A good death. An important aim for health services and for us all. BMJ. 2000;320:129–30.

3. Kübler-Ross E. On death and dying. London: Routledge; 1969.

4. Perreault A, Fothergill-Bourbonnais F, Fiset V. The experience of family members caring for a dying loved one. Int J Palliat Nurs. 2004;10:133–43.

5. Taube AW. Home care of dying patients. In: McDonald N, Oneschuk D, Hagen N, Doyle D, editors. Palliative medicine. A case-based manual. 2nd ed. Oxford: Oxford University Press; 2005. p. 375–88.

6. Thomas K. Caring for the dying at home. Oxford: Radcliffe Medical Press; 2003.

7. National Health Service End of Life Care Programme. Preferred priorites for care. Available at www.endoflifecareforadults.nhs.uk/tools/core-tools/preferredprioritiesforcare. Last accessed 27 Nov 2011.

8. Mack JW, Weeks JC, Wright AA, et al. End-of-life discussions, goal attainment, and distress at the end of life: predictors and outcomes of receipt of care consistent with preferences. J Clin Oncol. 2010;28:1203–8.

9. Ellershaw J, Wilkinson S, editors. Care of the dying. A pathway to excellence. Oxford: Oxford University Press; 2003.

10. National Institute for Clinical Excellence. Improving supportive and palliative care for adults with cancer. London: NICE; 2004.

11. Marie Curie Palliative Care Institute Liverpool. The liverpool care pathway for the dying patient LCP core documentation. Available at www.mcpcil.org.uk/liverpool-care-pathway/documentation-lcp.htm. Last accessed 27 Nov 2011.

12. Office of National Statistics. Mortality Statistics. 2004. Available at www.statistics.gov.uk/hub/population/deaths/mortality-rates/index.html. Last accessed 27 Nov 2011.

13. Department of Health. End of life care strategy. Available at www.dh.gov.uk/prod-con-sum_dh/groups/dh_digitalassets/@dh/@en/documents/digitalasset/dh_086345.pdf. Last accessed 27 Nov 2011.

14. Department of Social Services. What to do after a death in England or Wales. Available at www.dwp.gov.uk/docs/dwp1027.pdf. Last accessed 27 Nov 2011.

15. Scottish Government. What to do after a death in Scotland. Available at www.scotland.gov.uk/Resource/Doc/277028/0083194.pdf. Last accessed 27 Nov 2011.

16. Ministry of Justice. Cremation regulations 2008 guidance for cremation authorities and crematorium managers. 2008. Available at www.justice.gov.uk/guidance/docs/cremation-crematorium-guidance.pdf. Last accessed 27 Nov 2011.

17. Ministry of Justice. A guide to coroners and inquests. 2010. Available at www.direct.gov.uk/prod_consum_dg/groups/dg_digitalassets/@dg/@en/documents/digitalasset/dg_185904.pdf. Last accessed 27 Nov 2011.

18. Egan KA, Arnold RL. Grief and bereavement care. Am J Nurs. 2003;103:42–52.

19. Parkes CM. Coping with loss: consequences and implications for care. Int J Palliat Nurs. 1998;5:250–4.

20. Worden JW. Grief counselling and grief therapy. A handbook for the mental health practitioner. 4th ed. New York: Springer Publishing Co; 2009.

Chapter 7

Ethical Issues

Ethics are the principles that should guide clinicians in their work and decision-making. They apply to all medical care but assume greater importance when caring for people at the end of life. Unlike cultural issues, which differ from country to country, the same ethical principles apply everywhere. There are four main principles of medical ethics (Figure 7.1) [1].

Ethical dilemmas are situations arising when equally compelling ethical reasons both for and against a particular course of action are recognized and a decision must be made.

Ethical difference/conflict involves value preferences and arises where people of good will are uncertain of or disagree about the right thing to do when someone's life, health, or wellbeing is threatened by disease or illness. The following section outlines selected ethical issues in a palliative care setting.

Confidentiality

Confidentiality is an essential requirement for the preservation of trust between patients and healthcare professionals, and is subject to legal and ethical safeguards. Patients should be able to expect that information about their health, which they give in confidence, will be kept confidential unless there is a compelling reason why it should not. There is also a strong public interest in maintaining confidentiality so that individuals

G. Zeppetella, *Palliative Care in Clinical Practice,*
DOI 10.1007/978-1-4471-2843-4_7,
© Springer-Verlag London 2012

Four ethical principles

Autonomy	Respect for a	Treatments can be given only with patients' informed consent
		It is the patient's right to decide what treatments they do or do not wish to have
		Patients have a right to be fully informed in order to make decisions
		Healthcare professionals have an obligation to provide honest and complete information when it is requested
		Applies not only to medical treatments but also to matters such as where they receive care and who shall provide their care
Beneficence	Doing good for the patient	Whatever is done or said must be for the patient's good Includes being honest with patients, which in nearly all circumstances will be of benefit to the patients
		Patients should not be subjected to unnecessary investigations
		Patients should not be subjected to unnecessary or futile therapies
		Applies not only to physical good but also to psychological, social, and existential wellbeing Must be distinguished from paternalism
Non-malfeasance	Avoiding doing harm to the patient	Whatever is done or said must not harm the patient, physically or psychologically
		Includes being honest with patients; lying to patients or telling only part of the truth will very probably cause harm
		For every intervention, the potential benefits must be weighed against possible adverse effects
		Treatments should not be prescribed unless there is a strong chance that they will help the patient and have only a small chance of unpleasant adverse effects
Justice	Fair use of resources and equality of approach	Not according to wealth, class, creed, or color
		Unfortunately, observation of healthcare around the world shows much lack of justice
		Many treatments are only available to the rich, or those with influence and power, or those articulate enough to ask for something better
		In some countries morphine is available only if the patient can afford it
		In some countries even palliative care has to be paid for and lack of money may mean dying in pain, possibly alone, without any dignity

Figure 7.1 Four ethical principles. (Data from Doyle and Woodruff [1])

will be encouraged to seek appropriate treatment and share information relevant to it.

All identifiable patient information, whether written, computerized, visually, or audio recorded, or simply held in the memory of healthcare professionals, is subject to the duty of confidentiality. It covers the following:

- any clinical information about an individual's diagnosis or treatment
- a picture, photograph, video, audiotape, or other images of the patient
- who the patient's doctor is and what clinics patients attend and when
- anything else that may be used to identify patients either directly or indirectly so that any of the information above, combined with the patient's name or address or full postcode or the patient's date of birth, can identify them.

A doctor's duty of confidentiality is outlined by the UK General Medical Council [2].

From time to time, the duty to preserve confidentiality can present healthcare professionals with an ethical or legal dilemma, commonly when a third party requests information about patients or their treatment. A number of factors must be considered including the following:

- Patients must be properly informed as to how identifiable information about them is used.
- Data should be anonymized wherever possible.
- Explicit consent should be sought for the use or disclosure of personal health information, unless it is clearly implied.
- Occasionally, when it is not practicable to obtain consent, information may be disclosed where the law requires or where there is an overriding public interest, e.g., where child abuse is suspected.
- Disclosures should be kept to the minimum necessary to achieve the purpose.
- When patients withhold consent to disclosure of their information, their wishes should be respected.
- Healthcare professionals must always be prepared to justify their decisions about the use of personal health information.

Exceptions to confidentiality

- With patient consent
- For legal demand
- When judged to be in the patient's interest
- For registration of illness
- To protect society

Figure 7.2 Exceptions to confidentiality. (Data from the General Medical Council [2])

The duty of confidentiality extends to all members of the clinical team who require access to the patient's notes. In community settings many integrated teams have been established, which include workers from health, social services, and non-statutory bodies. Healthcare professionals should from the outset discuss with patients the desirability of sharing information with other agencies where appropriate. Other agencies may wish to be involved in discussions about patients at various points in their treatment or to attend case conferences or multidisciplinary meetings. In all these circumstances confidential information should be shared with explicit consent or, in the absence of consent, where disclosure is required by law or there is an overriding public interest in disclosure (Figure 7.2) [2].

Consent

Before undertaking any examination or investigation, providing treatment or involving patients in teaching or research, the clinician must be satisfied that they have consent or other valid authority. Usually this will involve providing information to patients in a way that they can understand, before asking for their consent.

In obtaining consent assumptions should not be made about:

- the information that a patient might want or need,
- the clinical or other factors that a patient might consider significant, and
- a patient's level of knowledge or understanding of what is proposed.

It is the responsibility of the clinician undertaking an investigation or providing treatment to discuss it with the patient. If this is not practical, the responsibility can be delegated to someone else, provided that they are suitably trained and qualified, have sufficient knowledge of the proposed investigation or treatment, and understand the risks involved and the principles of consent.

Patients can give consent orally or in writing, or they may imply consent by complying with the proposed examination or treatment, for example. In the case of minor or routine investigations or treatments, if the clinician is satisfied that the patient understands what is proposed and why, it is usually enough to have oral or implied consent. In cases that involve higher risk, it is important that the clinician obtains the patient's written consent.

Before accepting patients' consents, clinicians must consider whether they have been given the information that they want or need, and how well they understand the details and implications of what is proposed (Figure 7.3) [3].

Information necessary for making decisions should not be withheld for any other reason, including when a relative, partner, friend, or carer asks you to, unless the clinician believes that giving it would cause the

Information patients may want or need to provide consent

- The diagnosis and prognosis
- Any uncertainties about the diagnosis or prognosis, including options for further investigations
- Options for treating or managing the condition, including the option not to treat
- The purpose of any proposed investigation or treatment and what it will involve
- The potential benefits, risks, and burdens, and the likelihood of success, for each option; this should include information, if available, about whether the benefits or risks are affected by which organization or doctor is chosen to provide care
- Whether a proposed investigation or treatment is part of a research program or is an innovative treatment designed specifically for their benefit
- The people who will be mainly responsible for and involved in their care, what their roles are, and to what extent students may be involved
- Their right to refuse to take part in teaching or research
- Their right to seek a second opinion
- Any bills that they will have to pay
- Any conflicts of interest that you, or your organization, may have
- Any treatments that you believe have greater potential benefit for the patient than those that you or your organization can offer

Figure 7.3 Information patients may want or need to provide consent. (Data from the General Medical Council [3])

patient serious harm. In this context 'serious harm' means more than that the patient might become upset or decide to refuse treatment.

The clinician must respect a patient's decision to refuse an investigation or treatment, even if it is felt that the decision is wrong or irrational. Concerns about the possible consequences of the decision should be outlined and clearly explained but no pressure should be put on the patient to accept the advice. The patient's medical records or consent form should be used to record the key elements of the discussion with the patient irrespective of the outcome.

No one else can make a decision on behalf of an adult who has capacity. If patients ask clinicians to make decisions on their behalf or want to leave decisions to a relative, partner, friend, carer, or another person close to them, it is still important that the patient understands the options open to them, and what the treatment will involve. If they do not want this information, clinicians should try to find out why. If, after discussion, patients still do not want to know in detail about their condition or the treatment, clinicians should respect their wishes. The fact that a patient has declined this information should be recorded. It should be made clear that patients can change their mind and have more information at any time [3].

Request for and Refusal of Treatment

While competent, people generally decide their best interests for themselves, and they may sometimes request or decline certain procedures. Requests for positive interventions should be taken into account, but ultimately clinicians have to decide which options are clinically appropriate to offer. Patients or their families cannot insist upon clinically inappropriate treatment.

Regular dialogue to agree the goals of care will help empower the patient, family, and healthcare team, and provide clarity about treatment choices (Figure 7.4) [4]. The goals are dynamic and will evolve and be refined as the illness progresses.

In terms of treatment refusal, the law and codes of ethical practice emphasize that adults with mental capacity can refuse medical treatment, including life-prolonging procedures. Where adults refuse

An approach to formulating the goals of care and treatment plans

Consider the patient's experience of the illness

- Symptoms
- Suffering

Consider the illness

- Nature and status
- Likely course
- Medical options
- Nearness of death

Consider the patient as a person

- Wishes
- Goals
- Plans
- Hopes

Patient and family

Formulate the goals of care

- General
- Specific

Healthcare team

Consider possible treatments

- Burdens and benefits?
- Consistent with goals?

Figure 7.4 An approach to formulating the goals of care and treatment plans. (Data from Latimer [4]. © 1991, Elsevier)

treatment likely to benefit them, health professionals should ensure that there is no misunderstanding and provide information in a sensitive manner about the implications of refusal [5].

When assessing the applicability of advance refusals the following considerations apply [6]:

- whether the decision is clearly applicable to the patient's current circumstances,
- whether the decision specifies particular circumstances in which the refusal of treatment should not apply,
- how long ago the decision was made and whether it has been reviewed or updated (this may also be a factor in assessing validity), and
- whether there are reasonable grounds for believing that circumstances exist that the patient did not anticipate and that would have affected the decision if anticipated, e.g., any relevant clinical developments or changes in the patient's personal circumstances since the decision was made.

Good communication is essential and may include an exploration of alternative treatment options that might be acceptable to the individual. Ultimately, however, a refusal made by an adult with mental capacity must be respected.

Each occasion of a patient's expressed refusal should be documented in the medical record. Any limits or conditions that a patient may set on a refusal should also be clearly documented in the medical record.

Withholding and Withdrawing Medical Treatment

Medical treatment can legally and ethically be withdrawn when it is unable to benefit the patient, for example, when it is not in the patient's best interest, or if the patient has refused it. In practice, however, this can sometimes be a difficult decision. The guiding principles must be to protect the dignity, comfort, and rights of the patient, and to take into account any known wishes of the patient and the views of people close to patients who lack capacity [5].

Providing artificial nutrition and hydration (ANH) by intravenous feeding, and feeding by nasogastric tube, percutaneous endoscopic gastrostomy, and radiologically inserted gastrostomy feeding tubes, may provide symptom relief, or prolong or improve the quality of the patient's life. However, the current evidence about the benefits, burdens, and risks of these techniques as patients approach end of life is not clear cut [6]. This can lead to concerns that patients who are unconscious or semiconscious may be experiencing distressing symptoms and complications, or otherwise be suffering either because their needs for nutrition or hydration are not being met or because attempts to meet their perceived needs for nutrition or hydration may be causing them avoidable suffering [6].

The patient's nutrition and hydration needs should be assessed separately. If the assessment is that the provision of clinically assisted nutrition or hydration would not be of overall benefit to the patient, treatment should not be started at that time or should be withdrawn. The reasons should be explained to the patient, if appropriate, and those close to him or her, and any questions or concerns expressed responded to [6].

ANH are regarded in law as medical treatment, and should be treated in the same way as other medical interventions. Nevertheless, some people see nutrition and hydration, whether taken orally or by tube or drip, as part of basic nurture. For this reason it is especially important to listen and consider the views of the patient and of those close to them (including their cultural and religious views) and explain the issues to be considered, including the benefits, burdens, and risks of providing clinically assisted nutrition and hydration [6].

A second clinical opinion should be sought before ANH treatment is withdrawn or withheld from a patient who is not imminently dying. Furthermore, in England, Wales, and Northern Ireland, the withdrawal or withholding of ANH from a patient in a persistent vegetative state needs to be subject to court review [6].

If a consensus is reached that clinically assisted nutrition or hydration would not be of overall benefit to the patient and the treatment is withdrawn or not started, it should be ensured that the patient is kept comfortable and any distressing symptoms are addressed. The patient's condition should be monitored and the clinical team prepared to reassess the benefits, burdens, and risks of providing clinically assisted nutrition or hydration in light of changes in their condition [6].

Cardiopulmonary Resuscitation

When someone suffers a sudden cardiac or respiratory arrest, cardiopulmonary resuscitation (CPR) attempts to restart their heart or breathing and restore their circulation. If attempted promptly, CPR has a reasonable success rate in some circumstances. Generally, however, CPR has a very low success rate and the burdens and risks of CPR include harmful side effects such as rib fracture and damage to internal organs, adverse clinical outcomes such as hypoxic brain damage, and other consequences for the patient such as increased physical disability [6].

If cardiac or respiratory arrest is an expected part of the dying process and CPR will not be successful, making and recording an advance decision not to attempt CPR will help to ensure that the patient dies in a dignified and peaceful manner [7]. It may also help to ensure that the patient's last hours or days are spent in their preferred place of care by, for example, avoiding emergency admission from a community setting to hospital. These management plans are called "do not attempt CPR"

(DNACPR) orders, or "do not attempt resuscitation" or "allow natural death" decisions.

Decisions about whether CPR should be attempted must be based on the circumstances and the wishes of the individual patient, and may involve discussions with the patient or with those close to them (or both), as well as members of the healthcare team (Figure 7.4) [4]. Some patients

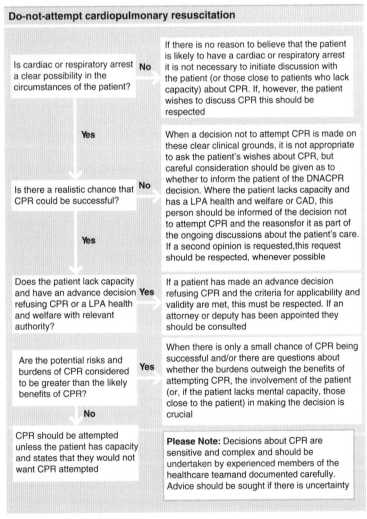

Figure 7.5 Do-not-attempt cardiopulmonary resuscitation (Continued overleaf)

with the capacity to make their own decisions may wish to refuse CPR. However, it can be difficult to establish patients' wishes and obtain relevant information about their underlying condition in order to make a considered judgment at the time they suffer a cardiac or respiratory arrest, and an urgent decision has to be made. So, if a patient has an existing condition that makes cardiac or respiratory arrest likely, establishing a management plan in advance will help to ensure that the patient's wishes and preferences about treatment can be taken into account and that, if appropriate, a DNACPR decision is made and recorded (Figure 7.5) [8].

Although some patients may want to be told, others may find discussion about interventions that would not be clinically appropriate burdensome and of little or no value. Information should not be withheld simply because conveying it is difficult or uncomfortable for the healthcare team. If patients do not wish to know about or discuss a DNACPR decision, their agreement to share with those close to them should be sought. Any discussions with patients, or with those close to them, about whether to attempt CPR, and any decisions made, should be documented in patients' records or ACPs [6].

It must be made clear to patients, to those close to them, and to members of the healthcare team that a DNACPR decision applies only to CPR. It does not imply that other treatments will be stopped or withheld. Other treatment and care will be provided if it is clinically appropriate and agreed to by a patient with capacity, or if it is of overall benefit to a patient who lacks capacity [6].

Euthanasia

Euthanasia (which comes from the Greek 'good death') is the active and intentional termination of a person's life. Euthanasia remains illegal in the UK.

Definitions

Euthanasia can be defined in numerous ways [9]:

- Voluntary euthanasia is when the person who is killed has requested to be killed.

Do-not-attempt cardiopulmonary resuscitation (continued)

Adults aged 16 years and over.
In the event of cardiac or respiratory arrest do not attempt cardiopulmonary resuscitation (CPR). All other appropriate treatment and care will be provided

Date of DNACPR order: _____ /_____ /_____

Name: _____

Address: _____

Date of birth: _____ /_____ /_____   NHS number: _____

Reason for DNACPR decision (tick one or more boxes and provide further information)

☐ CPR is unlikely to be successful [ie, medically futile] because: _____

_____

☐ Successful CPR likely to result in a length and quality of life not in the best interests of the patient because: _____

☐ Patient does not want to be resuscitated as evidenced by: _____

_____

Record of discussion of decision (tick one or more boxes and provide further information)

Discussed with the patient / Lasting Power of Attorney [welfare]?   ☐Yes ☐No

If 'yes' record content of discussion. If 'no' say why not discussed: _____

_____

Discussed with relatives/carers/others?   ☐Yes ☐No

If 'yes' record name, relationship to patient and content of discussion. If 'no' say why not discussed:

Discussed with other members of the health care team?   ☐Yes ☐No

If 'yes' record name, role and content of discussion. If 'no' say why not discussed: _____

Healthcare professional completing this DNACPR order

Name: _____

Signature: _____

Position: _____

Date: _____ /_____ /_____   Time: _____

Review and endorsement by responsible senior clinician

Name: _____

Signature: _____

Position: _____

Date: _____ _____ _____   Time: _____

Is DNACPR decision indefinite? ☐Yes ☐No

If 'no' specify review date: _____ /_____ /_____

Figure 7.5 Do-not-attempt cardiopulmonary resuscitation (continued). *CAD* Court Appointed Deputy, *DNACPR* do-not-attempt cardiopulmonary resuscitation, *LPA* Lasting Power of Attorney (Reproduced with permission from the East of England DNACPR Steering Group [8])

- Non-voluntary euthanasia is when the person who is killed made no request and gave no consent.
- Involuntary euthanasia is when the person who is killed made an expressed wish to the contrary.
- Assisted suicide: in this case, someone provides an individual with the information, guidance, and means to take his or her own life with the intention that they will be used for this purpose.
- Physician-assisted suicide: this is when a doctor helps another person to kill him- or herself.
- Euthanasia by action: this is intentionally causing a person's death by performing an action such as giving a lethal injection.
- Euthanasia by omission: this is intentionally causing death by not providing necessary and ordinary (usual and customary) care or food and water.

Physician-Assisted Suicide

Aiding or abetting suicide is also illegal and carries a potential 14-year prison sentence in the UK. The arguments for and against assisted suicide and physician-assisted suicide are similar to those made in relation to euthanasia. Assisted suicide differs from euthanasia in that the individual retains control of the process, rather than the doctor or anyone else assisting [5].

Euthanasia is not any of the following:
- not commencing treatment that would not provide a benefit to the patient,
- withdrawing treatment that has been shown to be ineffective, too burdensome, or unwanted, or
- the giving of high doses of analgesics that may endanger life, when they have been shown to be necessary.

The principle of 'double effect' is often cited to justify the third point (Figure 7.6) [10], although it is argued that we are responsible for all the anticipated consequences of our actions and that the intention is irrelevant.

Being confronted with requests for euthanasia has often been a source of concern for clinicians. The request is likely to be a reflection of the

Factors involved in the doctrine of double effect	
The good result must be achieved independently of the bad one	The unwanted result must not be the means of achieving the desired one, ie, the only way that the drug relieves the patient's pain is by death
The action must be proportional to the cause	The patient should not be given a dose of drugs far greater than required to control the symptom and certain to kill him or her
The action must be appropriate	The treatment given should be appropriate for the presenting symptoms
The patient must be in a terminal condition	Patients should not be given a potentially harmful dose of drug when they are likely to recover

Figure 7.6 **Factors involved in the doctrine of double effect**. (Data from the BBC [10])

patient's views and fears towards being ill, the physical, social, psychological, and spiritual pain, the possible deterioration that can come, and the hopeless nature of the situation. Each euthanasia request must therefore be open to discussion and, to this end, the following questions should be posed [11]:

• What motivation lies at the ground of the request for euthanasia? Is this really a request to actively put an end to life, or is the patient asking for caring guidance in the last days or weeks of his or her life?

• Does the patient have sufficient information (e.g., diagnosis and prognosis) on which grounds he or she makes the request?

• Is the patient mentally competent at the moment when making the request?

• Has the patient discussed the euthanasia request with other people?

• Does the patient make the request voluntarily? Is there no question of any form of coercion or pressure?

Arguments for the legalization of euthanasia are generally based on arguments about competent individuals' rights to choose the manner of their death or about cases where medicine is unable to control distressing terminal symptoms [7]. Terminally ill people can have their quality of life severely compromised by physical conditions such as incontinence, nausea and vomiting, breathlessness, paralysis, and difficulty in swallowing. Psychological factors that cause people to think of euthanasia include depression, fearing loss of control or dignity, feeling a burden, or dislike of being dependent.

Although suicide or traveling abroad to receive assisted suicide is not illegal, facilitating suicide is a criminal offence. In such circumstances, doctors need to be aware of the possible legal implications of these, or any other actions that might be seen as encouraging or facilitating suicide. As yet, no doctor providing a report or any accompanying person has been prosecuted for helping patients to travel abroad to end their lives. Nevertheless, some people feel that more detailed legal guidance should be available [7].

Arguments against legalization often focus on practical points. If euthanasia were an option, there might be pressure for all seriously ill people to consider it even if they would not otherwise entertain such an idea. Health professionals explaining options for the management of terminal illness would have to include an explanation of assisted dying. Patients might feel obliged to choose it for the wrong reasons, if they were worried about being a burden, or concerned about the financial implications of a long terminal illness [7]. Legalization could generate anxiety for vulnerable, elderly, disabled, or very ill patients. Some key points include:

- voluntary euthanasia leads to involuntary euthanasia,
- euthanasia is wide open to abuse,
- euthanasia could profoundly damage the doctor–patient relationship, and
- suffering can be treated without euthanasia.

With advances in the care of patients with advanced disease there is increasing support for patients and their carers at the end of life, making it less likely that such patients suffer uncontrolled physical pain or discomfort. It is essential that expertise in palliative care continues to develop, particularly in non-cancer disease, and that this expertise is disseminated throughout the UK National Health Service.

The Mental Capacity Act

The Mental Capacity Act 2005, which covers England and Wales, provides a statutory framework for people who lack capacity to make decisions for themselves, or who have capacity and want to make preparations for a time when they may lack capacity in the future. It sets out who can make decisions, in which situations, and how they should go about doing this.

The Act is intended to assist and support people who may lack capacity and to discourage anyone who is involved in caring for someone who lacks capacity from being overly restrictive or controlling. The term 'a person who lacks capacity' is intended to mean a person who lacks capacity to make a particular decision or take a particular action for him- or herself at the time that the decision or action needs to be taken.

Every adult has the right to make his or her own decisions if he or she has the capacity to do so. Family carers and healthcare or social care staff must assume that a person has the capacity to make decisions, unless it can be established that the person does not have capacity. People should receive support to help them make their own decisions. Before concluding that individuals lack capacity to make a particular decision, it is important to take all possible steps to try to help them reach a decision themselves.

People have the right to make decisions that others might think are unwise. Such a person should not automatically be labeled as lacking the capacity to make a decision. Any act done for, or any decision made on behalf of, someone who lacks capacity must be in his or her best interests. Any act done for, or any decision made on behalf of, someone who lacks capacity should be an option that is less restrictive of his or her basic rights and freedoms – as long as it is still in his or her best interests.

The Mental Capacity Act (Figure 7.7) has a significant impact on palliative and end-of-life care. Some of the most important features are as follows:

- new statutory tests or checklists:
  - to assess capacity, and
  - to determine best interests
- an emphasis on the importance of person-centered care,
- a duty to consult next of kin about relative's best interests,
- people's wishes and priorities must be taken into account when assessing their best interests, which means that ACP cannot be ignored,
- a new framework for advance decisions to refuse treatment,

Examples of situations in which the Mental Capacity Act may apply

- People living with dementia
- People living with impaired cognitive function
- People living with learning disability
- People living with severe psychiatric disorders
- Older people experiencing frailty
- People who are experiencing delirium or confusion
- People with fluctuating capacity or consciousness
- People on medication which causes persistent, transient, or fluctuating cognitive impairment
- People who are imminently dying and who no longer have full mental capacity
- People who are unconscious

Figure 7.7 Examples of situations in which the Mental Capacity Act may apply

- new proxy decision-making under lasting powers of attorney or when deputies are appointed by the court to make decisions,
- new advocacy in some cases – independent mental capacity advocates:
  - there is a Code of Practice, which professional carers must have regard to,
  - there is a new Court of Protection and Office of the Public Guardian,
  - there are two new criminal offences: willful neglect and ill treatment.

For further details visit: www.legislation.gov.uk/ukpga/2005/9/contents.

Advance Decisions

The Mental Capacity Act 2005 came into force in April 2007 and forms the legal basis for advance decisions. An advance decision (also called an advance directive) is used to indicate refusal of all or some forms of medical treatment if mental capacity is lost. It cannot be used to request treatment. A valid advance decision has the same effect as a refusal of treatment by a person with capacity: the treatment cannot lawfully be given – if it were, the doctor might face civil liability or criminal prosecution.

An advance decision cannot be used to:

- ask for life to be ended,
- force doctors to act against their professional judgment, or
- nominate someone else to decide about treatment on your behalf.

Valid Advance Decisions

To be valid an advance decision needs to:

- be made by a person who is 18 or over and has the capacity to make it,
- specify the treatment to be refused (it can do this in lay terms),
- specify the circumstances in which this refusal would apply,
- not have been made under the influence or harassment of anyone else, and
- not have been modified verbally or in writing since it was made.

Refusal of Life-Sustaining Treatment

Advance decisions refusing life-sustaining treatment must:

- be in writing (it can be written by a family member, recorded in medical notes by a doctor, or on an electronic record)
- be signed and witnessed (it can be signed by someone else at the person's direction – the witness is to confirm the signature, not the content of the advance directive)
- include an express statement that the decision stands "even if life is at risk."

When Might an Advance Decision Not Be Followed?

A doctor might not act on an advance decision for the following reasons:

- the person has done anything clearly inconsistent with the advance decision, which affects its validity (e.g., a change in religious faith)
- the current circumstances would not have been anticipated by the person and would have affected their decision (e.g., a recent development in treatment that radically changes the outlook for their particular condition)
- it is not clear about what should happen
- the person has been treated under the Mental Health Act.

A doctor can also treat if there is doubt or a dispute about the validity of an advance decision and the case has been referred to the court.

An advance statement is a general statement of a patient's wishes and views. It allows patients to state preferences and indicate what treatment or care they would like to receive if they are unable to decide or communicate their wishes. It can include non-clinical care including food preferences or whether they would prefer a bath to a shower. It could reflect religious or other beliefs and any aspects of life that they particularly value.

Only an advance decision is legally binding, but an advance statement should be taken into account when deciding what is in your best interests.

References

1. Doyle D, Woodruff R. The IAHPC manual of palliative care. 2nd ed. Houston: IAHPC Press; 2008. Available at: www.hospicecare.com/manual/IAHPCmanual.htm. Last accessed 27 Nov 2011.
2. General Medical Council. Guidance for doctors: confidentiality. 2009. Available at: www.gmc-uk.org/Confidentiality_core_2009.pdf_27494212.pdf. Last accessed 27 Nov 2011.
3. General Medical Council. Guidance for doctors: consent; patients and doctors making decisions together. 2008. Available at: www.gmc-uk.org/static/documents/content/Consent_0510.pdf. Last accessed 27 Nov 2011.
4. Latimer EJ. Ethical decision-making in the care of the dying and its applications to clinical practice. J Pain Symptom Manage. 1991;6:329–36.
5. BMA Ethics. End-of-life decisions. Views of the BMA. 2009. Available at: www.bma.org.uk/images/endlifedecisionsaug2009_tcm41-190116.pdf. Last accessed 27 Nov 2011.
6. General Medical Council. Guidance for doctors: treatment and care towards the end of life: good practice in decision making end of life. Available at: www.gmc-uk.org/static/documents/content/End_of_life.pdf. Last accessed 27 Nov 2011.
7. British Medical Association. Decisions relating to cardiopulmonary resuscitation. A joint statement from the British Medical Association, the Resuscitation Council (UK) and the Royal College of Nursing. 2007. Available at: www.bma.org.uk/images/DecisionsRelatingResusReport_tcm41-147300.pdf. Last accessed 27 Nov 2011.
8. East of England DNACPR Steering Group. DNACPR form. Available at: www.eoe.nhs.uk/page.php?page_id=2168. Last accessed 27 Nov 2011.
9. National Right to Life. Definitions. 2011. Available at. www.nrlc.org/euthanasia/index.html. Last accessed 27 Nov 2011.
10. BBC. The doctrine of double effect. Available at: www.bbc.co.uk/ethics/euthanasia/overview/doubleeffect.shtml. Last accessed 27 Nov 2011.
11. Gastmans C, Van Neste F, Schotsmans P. Facing requests for euthanasia: a clinical practice guideline. J Med Ethics. 2004;30:212–7.

Chapter 8

Prescribing in Palliative Care

The aim of drug therapy is to control symptoms in order that quality of life can be improved. The drug regimen should not become an unbearable burden for patients and carers or provoke unacceptable adverse effects (Figure 8.1). As patients are often polysymptomatic and require several drugs to control all their symptoms, the balance of benefit and detriment can be difficult to achieve because the resulting polypharmacy increases the risks of adverse effects, drug interactions, and non-adherence.

The General Principles of Prescribing in Palliative Care

The general principles of prescribing in palliative care include following:

- evaluation: diagnose the cause of symptoms (disease process, treatment adverse effects, general debility, and concurrent disorders)
- explanation: give a good and clear explanation of the mechanism underlying the symptom and treatment options, and involve caregivers
- individualized treatment: the patient should determine treatment priorities. Set realistic goals of treatment together
- supervision: regular reassessments should be made in order to ensure that dosage is optimum and to avoid unacceptable adverse effects.

G. Zeppetella, *Palliative Care in Clinical Practice*,
DOI 10.1007/978-1-4471-2843-4_8,
© Springer-Verlag London 2012

Pharmacotherapy: points to consider

- Diagnosis, including spread of disease
- Presence, frequency, and severity of symptoms, and impact on normal activities and sleep
- Drug history completed for all prescribed and purchased medicines
- Drug choice against local protocols and guidelines
- Anticipation of predictable side effects and prophylactic treatment initiated
- Patient's ability to take medicine in formulation prescribed
- Timely access to equipment to deliver medicine and appropriate training for professional caregiver, patient, and/or carer
- Patient's/carer's understanding of goals of therapy and potential side effects

Figure 8.1 Pharmacotherapy: points to consider

Benefits of medication review

- Identification, management, and prevention of adverse effects
- Ensure that patients have maximum benefit from their medicines
- Reduce the risk of drug-related problems
- Increase the appropriate use of medication
- Improve clinical outcomes
- Cost-effectiveness
- Increase quality of life
- Optimize therapy
- Reduce waste of medicines
- Enable patients to maintain their independence
- Reduce admissions to hospital
- Reduce drug-related deaths

Figure 8.2 Benefits of medication review. (Data from Wiffen et al. [1])

Medication Review

A regular medication review is required to maximize the therapeutic value and minimize the potential harm of the regimen (Figure 8.2) [1]. Medication review also gives patients an opportunity to discuss their medicines and any concerns that they might have, particularly as they are endeavoring to cope in an ever-changing situation.

Palliative Care Prescribing Issues

Important palliative care prescribing issues include the following:

- Prophylactic prescribing including around-the-clock medication for persistent symptoms; co-prescription of laxative and antiemetics with opioids to ensure optimum symptom relief.
- Simple, acceptable treatment regimens where the minimum possible number of drugs are prescribed, and size, shape, and taste of medication are considered along with the risk of adverse effects and drug interactions. Inconvenient doses or dose intervals should be avoided.
- A written advice chart is usually helpful for the patient and family to work from, with timings, names of drugs, and dose and purpose outlined.
- Continuity of care and communication are essential among all prescribers, nursing teams, and pharmacists, so all are aware of changes and the patient and family are not confused by medication changes. Availability of equipment (e.g., syringe drivers) and drugs needs to be assured, particularly out of hours, and changes in prescriptions should be anticipated to avoid delays in obtaining vital medication.
- Route of administration should be regularly reviewed. The oral administration can be limited by severe nausea or vomiting, dysphagia, bowel obstruction, weakness, or coma, and so is frequently not possible to the end of life; other options include rectal (e.g., morphine, oxycodone) or transdermal (fentanyl, buprenorphine) for background pain, and transmucosal fentanyl for breakthrough pain.
- Relative potencies can vary when switching between different opioids and different routes of administration; reassessment is mandatory.
- Unlicensed use of drugs commonly occurs in a palliative care setting and may involve the unlicensed use of drugs or the use of unlicensed routes.
- Progressive disease will alter how drugs are handled, particularly renal and hepatic failure.
- Individual differences exist between patients that may reflect age, use of adjuvant drug and non-drug measures, pharmacokinetic differences, pain tolerance threshold, previous use of strong opioids, duration of treatment, and adequacy of management of other symptoms.

Medication Adherence
Definitions

- Compliance is the term used to describe whether or not a patient takes the medication as directed. It implies little discussion between the healthcare professional and the patient.
- Concordance is a two-way exchange between the healthcare professional and patient. The patient participates in both the consultation and the decision-making process, and the patient's preferences and beliefs are taken into account.
- Adherence is somewhere between concordance and compliance. The healthcare professional accepts that the patient's beliefs, preferences, and prior knowledge influence medication taking and attempts to address this.

Prevalence

It is estimated that, on average, approximately 50% of patients on long-term therapy do not take their medication as directed. In a palliative care population the figure may be as high as 70% [2]. Non-adherence may take different forms:

- not filling a prescription,
- not taking medication,
- changes in dosage, timing, sequencing of administration, and
- taking of additional non-prescribed medication.

Assessment

A number of factors are reported to affect adherence (Figures 8.3 and 8.4) [3]. In many cases the cause may be involuntary (e.g., forgetting) or concerns about adverse effects.

Various methods of assessing adherence have been described, none of which is totally satisfactory.

General Management to Improve Adherence

Numerous strategies have been suggested:

- monitored dose systems,
- alarms,
- refill/follow-up reminders,

Factors reported to affect adherence

Ability to attend appointments	Gender
Age	Health beliefs and attitudes
Beliefs about medicines	Impact on daily life
Chaotic life style	Language
Complexity of regimen	Literacy
Concerns about confidentiality	Manual dexterity
Cost	Past or current experience of adverse effects
Cultural practices or beliefs	Satisfaction with healthcare
Depression	Self-esteem
Educational status	Adverse effects
Frequency of doses	Socioeconomic status

Figure 8.3 Factors reported to affect adherence. (Data from the World Health Organization [3])

The five dimensions of adherence

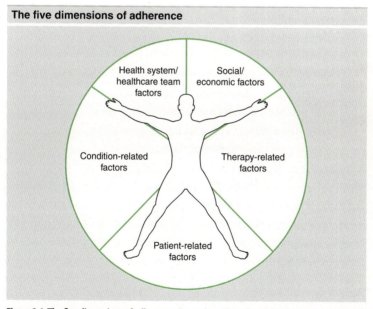

Figure 8.4 The five dimensions of adherence. (Reproduced from the World Health Organization [3])

- regimen simplification,
- written and oral patient information, and
- education programs.

Unlicensed Use of Medication

Once a new prescription drug has been approved, health professionals may discover that there are additional symptoms or conditions that the drug may treat effectively that were not among the reasons for the drug's original approval. A doctor may decide to prescribe the drug for one of these alternative reasons; such a prescription is considered to be beyond license or 'off-label.'

The use of drugs beyond license should be seen as a legitimate aspect of clinical practice that is both necessary and common. In palliative care, up to a quarter of all prescriptions are for drugs given for 'off-label' indications and/or via an unlicensed route [4]. Recommendations from bodies such as the General Medical Council in the UK place a duty on doctors to act responsibly, and to provide information to patients on the nature and associated risks of any treatment, including off-label and unlicensed drugs.

In the UK, a doctor may legally:

- Prescribe unlicensed medicines.
- Use unlicensed products specially prepared, imported, or supplied for a named patient.
- Use or advise using a licensed medicine for indications or in doses or by routes of administration outside the licensed recommendations.
- Supply another doctor with an unlicensed medicine.
- Override the warnings and precautions given in the license.
- Use unlicensed drugs in clinical trials.

Health professionals involved in prescribing, dispensing, and administering drugs beyond license should select those drugs that offer the best balance of benefit against harm for any given patient [5]. Where an unlicensed drug is prescribed, or the reasons for prescribing off-label are not well supported, the patient must be made aware of this. A detailed record should be kept of any drugs prescribed and the justification for their use.

Prescription of a drug (whether licensed use/route or not) requires the prescriber, in the light of published evidence, to balance both the potential good and the potential harm that might ensue. Prescribers have a duty to act with reasonable care and skill in a manner consistent with the practice of professional colleagues of similar standing. Thus, when prescribing outside the terms of the license, prescribers must be fully informed about the actions and uses of the drug, and be assured of the quality of the particular product.

Recommendations of the Association for Palliative Medicine and the British Pain Society

The following are the recommendations of the APM and the British Pain Society [5]:

- This statement should be seen as reflecting the views of a responsible body of opinion within the clinical specialties of palliative medicine and pain management.

- The use of drugs beyond license should be seen as a legitimate aspect of clinical practice.

- The use of drugs beyond license in palliative care and pain management practice is currently both necessary and common.

- Choice of treatment requires partnership between patients and healthcare professionals, and informed consent should be obtained, whenever possible, before prescribing any drug. Patients should be informed of any identifiable risks and details of any information given should be recorded. It is often unnecessary to take additional steps when recommending drugs beyond license.

- Patients, carers, and healthcare professionals need accurate, clear, and specific information that meets their needs. The APM and the Pain Society should work together with pharmaceutical companies to design accurate information for patients and their carers about the use of drugs beyond license.

- Health professionals involved in prescribing, dispensing, and administering drugs beyond license should select those drugs that offer the best balance of benefit against harm for any given patient.

- Health professionals should inform, change, and monitor their practice with regard to drugs used beyond license in the light of evidence from audit and published research.

- The Department of Health (UK) should work with health professionals and the pharmaceutical industry to enable and encourage the extension of product licenses where there is evidence of benefit in circumstances of defined clinical need.

- Organizations providing palliative care and pain management services should support therapeutic practices that are underpinned by evidence and advocated by a responsible body of professional opinion.
- There is an urgent need for the Department of Health to assist healthcare professionals to formulate national frameworks, guidelines, and standards for the use of drugs beyond license. The Pain Society and the APM should work with the Department of Health, NHS trusts, voluntary organizations, and the pharmaceutical industry to design accurate information for staff, patients, and their carers in clinical areas where drugs are used off-label. Practical support is necessary to facilitate and expedite surveillance and audit which are essential to develop this initiative.

Traveling Abroad with Controlled Drugs

With effect from January 1, 2008, persons traveling abroad (or visitors traveling to the UK) for longer than 3 months, or travelers carrying more than 3 months' supply of medication, are required to have a personal export or import license, as appropriate. This is a change from the previous regulation where a license was required if carrying opioids in excess of a defined amount. A personal license has no legal standing outside the UK and is intended to assist travelers passing through UK customs controls with their prescribed controlled drugs.

Travelers are advised to contact the embassy/consulate/high commission of the country of destination (or any country through which they may be traveling) regarding the local policy on the importation of controlled drugs.

Controlled drugs should be:

- carried in their original packaging,
- carried in hand luggage (BAA/airline regulations permitting),
- carried with a valid personal import/export license (if necessary), and
- carried with a letter from the prescribing doctor confirming the carrier's name, destination, drug details/amounts, unless a personal license is held.

For further details visit the relevant official government department.

Drugs in Special Circumstances
Prescribing in Hepatic Impairment

Liver disease may alter the response to drugs in several ways, and drug prescribing should be kept to a minimum in all patients with severe liver disease. The main problems occur in patients with jaundice, ascites, or evidence of encephalopathy [6].

Metabolism by the liver is the main route of elimination for many drugs, but hepatic reserve is large and liver disease has to be severe before important changes in drug metabolism occur. Routine LFTs are a poor guide to the capacity of the liver to metabolize drugs, and in the individual patient it is not possible to predict the extent to which the metabolism of a particular drug may be impaired [6].

A few drugs, e.g., rifampicin and fusidic acid, are excreted in the bile unchanged, and can accumulate in patients with intrahepatic or extrahepatic obstructive jaundice. The hypoalbuminemia in severe liver disease is associated with reduced protein binding and increased toxicity of some highly protein-bound drugs such as phenytoin and prednisolone. Reduced hepatic synthesis of blood-clotting factors, indicated by a prolonged prothrombin time, increases the sensitivity to oral anticoagulants such as warfarin and phenindione [6].

Hepatic Encephalopathy

In severe liver disease many drugs can further impair cerebral function and may precipitate hepatic encephalopathy. These include all sedative drugs, opioid analgesics, those diuretics that produce hypokalemia, and drugs that cause constipation. Edema and ascites in chronic liver disease can be exacerbated by drugs that give rise to fluid retention, e.g., NSAIDs and corticosteroids. Hepatotoxicity is either dose related or unpredictable (idiosyncratic). Drugs that cause dose-related toxicity may do so at lower doses in the presence of hepatic impairment than in individuals with normal liver function, and some drugs that produce reactions of the idiosyncratic kind do so more frequently in patients with liver disease. These drugs should be avoided or used very carefully in patients with liver disease [6].

Prescribing in Renal Impairment

The use of drugs in patients with reduced renal function can give rise to problems for several reasons [6]:

- reduced renal excretion of a drug or its metabolites may cause toxicity,
- sensitivity to some drugs is increased even if elimination is unimpaired,
- many side effects are tolerated poorly by patients with renal impairment, and
- some drugs are not effective when renal function is reduced.

Many of these problems can be avoided by reducing the dose or by using alternative drugs. It has been estimated that up to a third of patients with renal dysfunction also receive opioids. Most opioids are metabolized in the liver and excreted via the kidneys. In renal impairment, the parent compound and its metabolites may accumulate. Morphine, hydromorphone, and oxycodone may all be problematic in patients with renal impairment and, if used, will require careful monitoring.

Fentanyl, alfentanil, and methadone are considered relatively safe in renal failure because there are no active metabolites. Buprenorphine also appears relatively safe, although metabolites do accumulate in renal failure and a dose reduction may be necessary.

The level of renal function below which the dose of a drug must be reduced depends on the proportion of the drug eliminated by renal excretion and its toxicity. For many drugs with only minor or no dose-related side effects, a very precise modification of the dose regimen is unnecessary and a simple scheme for dose reduction is sufficient. For more toxic drugs with a small safety margin or patients at extremes of weight, dose regimens based on creatinine clearance should be used. When both efficacy and toxicity are closely related to plasma drug concentration, recommended regimens should be regarded only as a guide to initial treatment; subsequent doses must be adjusted according to clinical response and plasma drug concentration.

Renal function declines with age. Many elderly patients have renal impairment but, because of reduced muscle mass, this may not be indicated by a raised serum creatinine. It is wise to assume at least mild impairment of renal function when prescribing for elderly people [6].

The total daily maintenance dose of a drug can be reduced either by reducing the size of the individual doses or by increasing the interval between doses. For some drugs, although the size of the maintenance dose is reduced, it is important to give a loading dose if an immediate effect is required. This is because it takes about five times the half-life of the drug to achieve steady-state plasma concentrations. As the plasma half-life of drugs excreted by the kidney is prolonged in renal impairment, it can take many doses for the reduced dosage to achieve a therapeutic plasma concentration. The loading dose should usually be the same size as the initial dose for a patient with normal renal function [6].

Elderly Patients

Elderly patients often receive multiple drugs for their multiple diseases. This greatly increases the risk of drug interactions as well as adverse reactions, and may affect compliance. The balance of benefit and harm of some medicines may be altered in elderly people. They may also be more sensitive to many commonly used drugs, such as opioid analgesics, benzodiazepines, antipsychotics, and anti-parkinsonian drugs, all of which must be used with caution.

Elderly patients' medicines should be reviewed regularly and medicines that are not of benefit should be stopped. In some cases prophylactic drugs are inappropriate if they are likely to complicate existing treatment or introduce unnecessary side effects, especially in elderly patients with poor prognosis or with poor overall health (Figure 8.5) [6].

Patients with a History of Substance Abuse

The proportion of patients with cancer pain who are substance misusers is unknown, but likely reflects the general population. Patients with a current or past history of substance misuse are particularly challenging and opioid therapy is fundamentally no different from other patients with cancer pain, and should employ the basic principles of good pain control with the added consideration of the unique pharmacological needs of this patient group.

Guidance for medication use in elderly people

Limit range	It is a sensible policy to prescribe from a limited range of drugs and to be thoroughly familiar with their effects in elderly people
Reduce dose	Dosage should generally be substantially lower than for younger patients and it is common to start with about 50% of the adult dose. Some drugs (eg, long-acting anti-diabetic drugs such as glibenclamide) should be avoided altogether
Review regularly	Review repeat prescriptions regularly. In many patients it may be possible to stop some drugs, provided that clinical progress is monitored. It may be necessary to reduce the dose of some drugs as renal function declines
Simplify regimens	Elderly patients benefit from simple treatment regimens. Only drugs with a clear indication should be prescribed and whenever possible given once or twice daily. In particular, regimens that call for a confusing array of dosage intervals should be avoided
Explain clearly	Write full instructions on every prescription (including repeat prescriptions) so that containers can be properly labeled with full directions. Avoid imprecisions such as "as directed." Child-resistant containers may be unsuitable
Repeats and disposal	Instruct patients what to do when drugs run out, and also how to dispose of any that are no longer necessary. Try to prescribe matching quantities

Figure 8.5 Guidance for medication use in elderly people. (Data from the British National Formulary [6])

Prescribing for opioids for substance misusers

- Where possible choose a modified-release opioid
- Limit the use of normal-release opioids
- Maximize the use of adjuvant analgesics
- Maximize the use of non-pharmacological therapies
- Consider limiting the total dose dispensed at any one time
- Use pill counts and urine screening as necessary
- Liaise with the local substance misuse team

Figure 8.6 Prescribing for opioids for substance misusers. (Data from the British Pain Society [7])

It is important to complete a thorough substance use history and distinguish between those who are active misusers and those who are at risk or in recovery. The processes may be aided by explaining why this information is important and by being empathic and non-judgmental. A treatment plan should be formalized and coordinated with all other involved health professionals (Figure 8.6) [7]. Where possible, patient participation should be encouraged and the use of a written opioid agreement with carefully defined patient and provider expectations considered. Frequent and careful monitoring allows for close patient observation and prescription of limited quantities of opioids, and will usually distinguish whether deteriorating function is due to substance abuse or disease progression. It is important to recognize that substance misuse is often a chronic relapsing problem.

Opioids and Driving

Prescribers and other healthcare professionals should advise patients if treatment is likely to affect their ability to drive. This applies especially to drugs with sedative effects. Patients should be warned that these effects are increased by alcohol [6].

Cancer patients taking stable doses of appropriately titrated opioids have only a slight and selective effect on functions relating to driving. Thus, patients should be advised not to drive for a week after starting a regularly scheduled opioid, and a week after a dose increase, although the optimal interval between dose initiation or increase and returning to driving is unclear, and may vary between individuals and formulation used. It is also advisable to avoid driving after taking supplemental doses of opioids (Figure 8.7).

The General Medical Council guidelines state that doctors have a duty to inform patients when prescribing medication that may impair their driving, and that the patient has a legal duty to inform the Driver and Vehicle Licensing Agency (DVLA) of any circumstances that may render them unfit to drive. Although there is no legal obligation to do so, it is also appropriate to advise patients that motor insurance policies usually require patients to inform them of any change in their medical circumstances for the policy to remain valid.

General information about a patient's fitness to drive is available from the DVLA at www.dvla.gov.uk.

Opioids and driving: when not to drive

- Unless patient feels 100% safe to do so
- If patient feels tired or sleepy
- After taking any other sedative drug
- After drinking alcohol
- After taking extra doses of opioids (eg, for at least 3 h after an extra dose of morphine)
- After starting or increasing the dose of a opioid

Figure 8.7 Opioids and driving: when not to drive

Syringe Drivers

Successful pharmacotherapy often depends on the mode of drug delivery. Although the oral route is often preferred because it is convenient and usually inexpensive, there are circumstances when the oral route is neither feasible nor desirable. One such alternative is the CSCI via syringe driver.

There are a number of indications for CSCI in a palliative care setting (Figure 8.8), where the syringe driver allows for:

- increased comfort for the patient because there is less need for repeated injections,
- control of multiple symptoms with a combination of drugs,
- round-the-clock comfort because plasma drug concentrations are maintained without peaks and troughs,
- independence and mobility maintained because the device is lightweight and can be worn in a holster under or over clothes, and
- generally needs to be loaded only daily.

Two of the most common syringe drivers are the Graseby™ MS16 (Blue), set at millimeters per hour (i.e., with 48-mm infusion set at 2 mm/h) and the Graseby MS26 (Green), set at millimeters per day (i.e., with 48-mm infusion set at 48 mm/day) (Figure 8.9) [8]. Where possible, use local protocols for setting up a syringe driver (Figure 8.10).

Diamorphine has traditionally been the parenteral opioid of choice in the UK; however, other opioids can also be used:

- Diamorphine is very similar to morphine, but more soluble and more lipophilic, allowing it to cross the blood–brain barrier more easily. Clinically, the principal advantage of diamorphine over morphine is

Indications for considering a syringe driver
• Difficulty swallowing
• Oral or pharyngeal lesions
• Persistent nausea or vomiting
• Poor alimentary absorption
• Intestinal obstruction
• Profound weakness or cachexia
• Comatose or moribund patient

Figure 8.8 Indications for considering a syringe driver

Commonly used syringe drivers

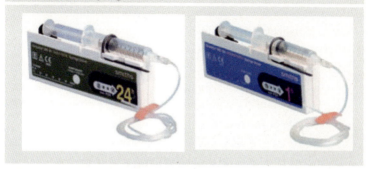

Figure 8.9 Commonly used syringe drivers. (Reproduced with permission from Medinor [8])

Setting up a syringe driver

- Calculate the 24-hour doses of medication to be delivered
- Draw up required drugs into the syringe with diluent
- Measure the contents of the syringe against the millimeter scale on the barrel
- Most drugs are mixed with 0.9% saline; notable exemptions are cyclizine and high concentrations of diamorphine when water for injection is preferred
- An infusion set is attached to the syringe
- Prime the line (this means the first infusion will last less than 24 hours)
- Labelsyringe with date, patient's name, contents, and sign
- Fit and secure the syringe to the driver with the black strap
- Site the needle subcutaneously (the upper chest and arm are commonly used)
- Press the start button and ensure that you hear a whirring sound and that the light flashes

Figure 8.10 Setting up a syringe driver

its greater solubility, which may be advantageous in subcutaneous administration. Hence, although oral preparations are available, it is principally the injection that is used. In the opioid-naïve patient the usual starting dose is 5–10 mg sc over 24 h. Supplemental doses during titration are roughly one-sixth of the total daily diamorphine dose delivered 4 hourly as required.

- Morphine may be delivered parentally. The average relative potency ratio of oral to intravenous morphine is between 1:2 and 1:3. In the opioid-naïve patient the usual starting dose is 10–20 mg sc over 24 h. Supplemental doses during titration are roughly one-sixth of the total daily morphine dose delivered 4 hourly as required.

- Alfentanil is a parenteral opioid analgesic commonly used as an intraoperative anesthetic agent, but that is of value in the management of pain in patients with renal failure. It is metabolized in the liver to inactive compounds and has a short half-life and short duration of action. In the opioid-naïve patient the usual starting dose is 0.5–1.0 mg sc over 24 h. Supplemental doses during titration are roughly one-sixth of the total daily alfentanil dose delivered 2 hourly as needed because of its short duration of action.
- Oxycodone may be delivered by either subcutaneous or intravenous injections or infusions. In the opioid-naïve patient, the usual starting dose is 5–10 mg sc over 24 h. Supplemental doses during titration are roughly one-sixth of the total daily oxycodone dose delivered 4 hourly as required.

Local guidelines are often available from palliative care units and should be sought, particularly when mixing drugs in a syringe driver. There are generally few compatibility problems with common two- and three-drug combinations containing [9]:

- diamorphine,
- oxycodone,
- alfentanil,
- morphine,
- haloperidol,
- metoclopramide,
- levomepromazine,
- hyoscine (scopolamine) hydrobromide, and
- midazolam.

However there can be problems with:

- cyclizine,
- hyoscine (scopolamine) butylbromide (Buscopan),
- ketorolac, and
- dexamethasone.

Syringe driver troubleshooting	
Problem	**Possible cause**
Driver not functioning	Flat battery Battery inserted incorrectly Blocked cannula Start button not pressed
Driver functioning but light not flashing **Alarm sounding**	Low battery Syringe empty Kinked tubing/cannula blocked Driver malfunction
Infusion too slow	Check site inflamed or cannula blocked Has tubing kinked? Are syringe and tubing still connected? Is syringe plunger accurately in place?
Infusion too fast	Check rate setting and calculation
Recurrenvt site inflammation	Review drugs Reduce concentration of irritant drug Change to alternative drug Switch to plastic cannula Add dexamethasone to mixture

Figure 8.11 Syringe driver troubleshooting

A syringe driver takes a few hours to establish a steady-state drug level in plasma, and therefore one should consider immediately subcutaneous injections of appropriate medication while setting the syringe driver up.

Regular checks on syringe driver operation must be built into the daily routine. In particular, one should look out for signs of precipitation in the syringe, and ensure that the rate of administration and the volume of drugs left in the syringe are correct. Furthermore, the integrity of the administration line, cannula, and syringe driver should be checked (Figure 8.11).

End-of-Life Care

Figures 8.12, 8.13, 8.14, 8.15, and 8.16 give examples of symptom algorithms used as part of the LCP in the management of common problems at the end of life [11]. Where possible it is advised that local guidance be sought. Where problems persist, despite following locally agreed algorithms, contact the specialist palliative care team.

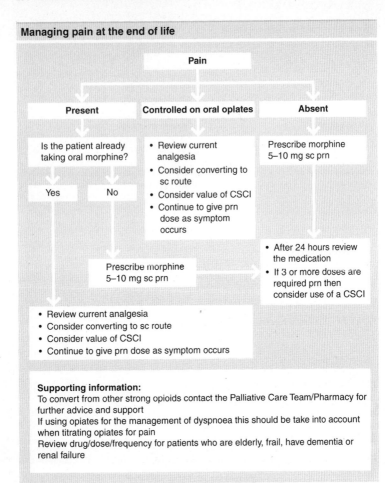

Figure 8.12 Managing pain at the end of life. (Reproduced with kind permission from the LCP Central Team at the Marie Curie Palliative Care Institute Liverpool [10])

Managing terminal restlessness and agitation

Agitation and restlessness

Present

Prescribe midazolam 2.5–5 mg sc prn

- After 24 hours review the medication
- If 3 or more doses are required prn then consider use of CSCI

Continue to give prn doses as symptom occurs

Absent

Prescribe midazolam 2.5–5 mg sc prn
Anticipatory prescribing in this manner will ensure that in the last hours or days of life there is no delay in responding to a symptom if it occurs

Supporting information:
The management of agitation and restlessness does not usually require the use of opioids unless the agitation and restlessness is thought to be caused by pain
Review drug/dose/frequency for patients who are elderly, frail, have dementia or renal failure

Figure 8.13 Managing terminal restlessness and agitation. (Reproduced with kind permission from the LCP Central Team at the Marie Curie Palliative Care Institute Liverpool [10])

Managing respiratory tract secretions

Respiratory tract secretions

Present	Absent
Prescribe hyoscine hydrobromide 400 μg sc	Prescribe hyoscine hydrobromide 400 μg sc
CSCI −1200 μg over 24 hours	Anticipatory prescribing in this manner will ensure that in the last hours or days of life there is no delay in responding to asymptom if it occurs
Continue to give prn dosage as symptom occurs	
If symptoms persist then after 24 hours consider increasing the total 24 hour dose to 2400 μg	

Supporting information:

Glycopyrronium 200 prn may be used as an alternative μg sc
Review drug/dose/frequency for patients who are elderly, frail, have dementia or renal failure

Figure 8.14 Managing respiratory tract secretions. (Reproduced with kind permission from the LCP Central Team at the Marie Curie Palliative Care Institute Liverpool [10])

Managing nausea and vomiting

Nausea and vomiting

Present

Prescribe cyclizine 50 mg sc TDS

- After 24 hours review the medication
- If 2 or more doses are required prn then consider cyclizine 150 mg via CSCI

Absent

Prescribe cyclizine 50 mg sc 8 hourly prn Anticipatory prescribing in this manner will ensure that in the last hours or days of life there is no delay in responding to a symptom if it occurs

Supporting information:

Always use water for the injection when making up cyclizine

Cyclizine is not recommended in patients with heart failure – seek advice and support

Alternative anti-emetics, may be prescribed eg:
- Haloperidol 1.5–3 mg sc prn (1.5–5 mg via a CSCI over 24 hrs – if required)
- Levomepromazine 6.25 mg sc prn (6.25–12.5 mg via CSCI over 24 hrs – if required)

Review drug/dose/frequency for patients who are elderly, frail, have dementia or renal failure

Figure 8.15 Managing nausea and vomiting. (Reproduced with kind permission from the LCP Central Team at the Marie Curie Palliative Care Institute Liverpool [10])

Managing dyspnea

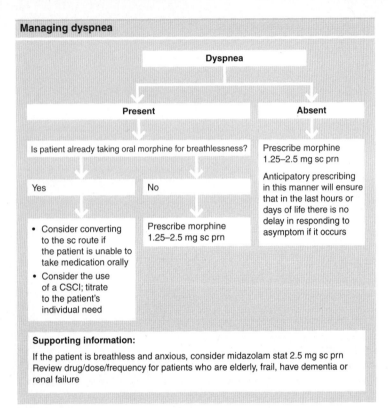

Figure 8.16 **Managing dyspnea**. (Reproduced with kind permission from the LCP Central Team at the Marie Curie Palliative Care Institute Liverpool [10])

References

1. Wiffen P, Mitchell M, Snelling M, Stoner N. Oxford handbook of clinical pharmacy. Oxford: Oxford University Press; 2007.
2. Zeppetella G. How do terminally ill patients at home take their medication? Palliat Med. 1999;13:469–75.
3. World Health Organization. Adherence to long-term therapies: evidence for action. Geneva: WHO; 2003.
4. Palliative Drugs. Using licensed drugs for unlicensed purposes. 2011. Available at: www.palliativedrugs.com/using-licensed-drugs-for-unlicensed-purposes. Last accessed 27 Nov 2011.
5. The British Pain Society. The use of drugs beyond licence in palliative care and pain management. 2005. Available at: www.britishpainsociety.org/book_usingdrugs_main.pdf. Last accessed 27 Nov 2011.
6. British National Formulary. BNF 61. London: BMJ Group and Pharmaceutical Press; 2011. Available at: www.bnf.org. Last accessed 27 Nov 2011.

7. British Pain Society. Pain and substance misuse: improving the patient experience. 2007. Available at: www.britishpainsociety.org/book_drug_misuse_main.pdf. Last accessed 27 Nov 2011.

8. Medinor. Infusjonspumpe. 2011. Available at: www.medinor.no/medinor7/frontend/ mediabank/1/15307/0105-0504-l.jpg. Last accessed 27 Nov 2011.

9. Dickman A, Schneider J, Varga J. The syringe driver: continuous subcutaneous infusions in palliative care. 2nd ed. Oxford: Oxford University Press; 2005.

10. Marie Curie Palliative Care Institute Liverpool. Medication guidance: symptom control algorithms. Available at: www.liv.ac.uk/mcpcil/liverpool-care-pathway/documentation-lcp. htm. Last accessed 14 Dec 2011.

11. Ellershaw J, Wilkinson S, editors. Care of the dying. A pathway to excellence. Oxford: Oxford University Press; 2003.

Further Reading

Charlton R. Primary palliative care: dying, death and bereavement in the community. Oxford: Radcliffe Medical Press; 2002.

Davies A, Finlay I. Oral care in advanced disease. Oxford: Oxford University Press; 2005.

Davies AN, Epstein JB. Oral complications of cancer and its management. Oxford: Oxford University Press; 2010.

Dickman A. Drugs in palliative care. Oxford: Oxford University Press; 2010.

Fallon M, Hanks G. ABC of palliative care. London: Blackwell Publishing; 2006.

Gagnon PR. Treatment of delirium in supportive and palliative care. Curr Opin Support Palliat Care. 2008;2:60–6.

Hanks G, Cherny N, Kaasa S, et al., editors. Oxford textbook of palliative medicine. 4th ed. Oxford: Oxford University Press; 2009.

Jeffrey D. Patient-centred ethics and communication at the end of life. Oxford: Radcliffe Publishing Limited; 2006.

G. Zeppetella, *Palliative Care in Clinical Practice*,
DOI 10.1007/978-1-4471-2843-4,
© Springer-Verlag London 2012

National Institute for Health and Clinical Excellence. Delirium. Diagnosis, prevention and management, NICE clinical guidelines 103. London: National Clinical Guideline Centre for Acute and Chronic Conditions; 2010.

National Institute for Health and Clinical Excellence. Depression. The treatment and management of depression in adults, NICE clinical guideline 90. London: National Collaborating Centre for Mental Health; 2009.

Sykes N, Edmonds P, Wiles J, editors. Management of advanced disease. 4th ed. London: Arnold; 2006.

Twycross R, Wilcock A, editors. Palliative care formulary. 3rd ed. Nottingham: Palliativedrugs.com Ltd; 2009.

Twycross R, Wilcock A, Stark Toller C. Symptom management in advanced cancer. 4th ed. Nottingham: Palliativedrugs.com Ltd; 2010.

Watson M, et al., editors. Oxford handbook of palliative care. Oxford: Oxford University Press; 2005.

Woodruff R. Palliative medicine. 4th ed. Oxford: Oxford University Press; 2004.

Worthington R, Stone P, Thorns A. Ethics and palliative care: a case-based manual. Oxford: Radcliffe Publishing Ltd; 2005.

Zeppetella G. Successful management of cancer pain. London: Evolving Medicine Ltd; 2010.

Zylicz Z, Twycross R, Jones A, editors. Pruritus in advanced disease. Oxford: Oxford University Press; 2004.

Useful Websites

Mental Capacity Act 2005 Code of practice. www.dca.gov.uk/Legal-policy/mental-capacity/mca-cp.pdf.

The National End of Life Care Programme. www.endoflifecareforadults.nhs.uk.

Preferred Priorities for Care. www.endoflifecareforadults.nhs.uk/tools/core-tools/preferredprioritiesforcare.

The Gold Standards Framework. www.goldstandardsframework.nhs.uk.

Macmillan Cancer Support. www.macmillan.org.uk.

Liverpool Care Pathway for the Dying Patient. www.mcpcil.org.uk/Liverpool-care-pathway.

The National Council for Palliative Care. www.ncpc.org.uk.

World Health Organization Palliative Care. www.who.int/cancer/palliative.

Palliative Drugs Website. www.palliativedrugs.com/compatibility-charts.

Hematology and Biochemistry

Hematology	
Test	**Normal range**
Hemoglobin (Hb)	13.0–18.0 g/day (male); 12.0–15.0 g/day (female)
White blood cell count	4.0–10.0 × 10⁹/L
Platelets	150–450 × 10⁹/L
Hematocrit (HCT)	Male: 41–50%; female: 35–46%
Mean cell volume (MCV)	83–101 fL
Mean cell hemoglobin (MCH)	27.0–32.0 pg
Mean cell hemoglobin concentration (MCHC)	31.5–34.5 g/dL
Red cell distribution width (RDW)	11.6–14.0%
Erythrocyte sedimentation rate (ESR)	<10
Prothrombin time (PTT)	11.5–13.9 s
International normalized ratio (INR)	2.0–4.5
Activated partial thromboplastin time (APTT)	21.0–32.0 s
Red blood cell count	3.80–4.80 × 10¹²/L
Neutrophils	2.0–7.0 × 10⁹/L
Lymphocytes	1.0–3.0 × 10⁹/L
Monocytes	0.2–1.0 × 10⁹/L
Eosinophils	0.0–0.5 × 10⁹/L
Basophils	0.00–0.01 × 10⁹/L

Biochemistry	
Test	Normal range
Sodium	135–148 mmol/L
Potassium	3.5–5.0 mmol/L
Creatinine	80–120 µmol/L (male); 60–105 µmol/L (female)
Urea	3.7–9.2 mmol/L
Calcium	2.12–2.55 mmol/L
Corrected calcium[a]	2.12–2.55 mmol/L
Alkaline phosphatase (ALP)	<115 IU/L
Total protein	62–76 g/L
Albumin	35–47 g/L
Globulin	23–35 g/L
Total bilirubin	5–16 µmol/L
Glucose fasting/random	Fasting: 3.5–5.5 mmol/L; random: <11 mmol/L
Alanine transaminase (AST)	<40 IU/L (male); <31 IU/L (female)

[a]Corrected calcium (mmol/L) = (40 serum albumin in g/l × 0.02

Appendix 2

Assessment Tools

The following are illustrated in this appendix:

- HADS (Figure A.2.1) [1],
- Distress thermometer (Figure A.2.2) [2],
- Abbreviated Mental Test Score (Figure A.2.3) [3],
- Brief Pain Inventory (Figure A.2.4) [4],
- Leeds Assessment of Neuropathic Symptoms and Signs (Figure A.2.5) [5],
- Dermatome map (Figure A.2.6) [6], and
- Breakthrough Pain Assessment Schedule (Figure A.2.7) [7].

Hospital Anxiety and Depression Scale

This questionnaire will help your physician know how you are feeling. Read every sentence. Place an "X" on the answer that best describes how you have been feeling during the LAST week. you do not have to think too much to answer. In this questionnaire, spontaneous answer are more important. Mark only one answer for each question.

A 1. I feel tense or wound up:

3 ☐ Most of the time		1 ☐ From time to time	
2 ☐ A lot of times		0 ☐ Not at all	

D 2. I still enjoy the things I used to:

0 ☐ Definitely as much		2 ☐ Only a little	
1 ☐ Not quite so much		3 ☐ Hardly at all	

A 3. I get a sort of frightened feeling as if something awful is about to happen:

3 ☐ Very definitely and quite badly		1 ☐ A little, but it doesn't worry me	
2 ☐ Yes, but not too badly		0 ☐ Not at all	

Figure A.2.1 Hospital Anxiety and Depression Scale (continued overleaf)

Hospital Anxiety and Depression Scale

This questionnaire will help your physician know how you are feeling. Read every sentence. Place an "X" on the answer that best describes how you have been feeling during the LAST WEEK. You do not have to think too much to answer. In this questionnaire, spontaneous answer are more important. Mark only one answer for each question.

D 4. I can laugh and see the funny side of things:

0 ☐ As much as I always could	2 ☐ Definitely not so much now
1 ☐ Not quite as much now	3 ☐ Not at all

D 5. Worrying thoughts go through my mind:

3 ☐ Most of the time	1 ☐ From time to time
2 ☐ A lot of times	0 ☐ Only occasionally

A 6. I feel cheerful:

0 ☐ Most of the time	2 ☐ Not often
1 ☐ Usually	3 ☐ Not at all

A 7. I can sit at ease and feel relaxed:

0 ☐ Definitely	2 ☐ Not often
1 ☐ Usually	3 ☐ Not at all

D 8. I feel as if I am slowed down:

3 ☐ Nearly all the time	1 ☐ From time to time
2 ☐ Very often	0 ☐ Not at all

A 9. I get a sort of frightened feeling like butterflies in the stomach:

0 ☐ Not at all	2 ☐ Quite often
1 ☐ From time to time	3 ☐ Very often

D 10. I have lost interest in my appearance:

3 ☐ Definitely	1 ☐ I may not take quite as much care
2 ☐ I don't take so much care as I should	0 ☐ I take just as much care as ever

A 11. I feel restless, as if I have to be on the move:

3 ☐ Very much indeed	1 ☐ Not very much
2 ☐ Quite a lot	0 ☐ Not at all

A 12. I look forward with enjoyment to things:

0 ☐ As much as I ever did	2 ☐ Definitely less than I used to
1 ☐ A little less than I used to	3 ☐ Hardly at all

A 13. I get a sudden feeling of panic:

3 ☐ Very often indeed	1 ☐ From time to time
2 ☐ Quite often	0 ☐ Not at all

A 14. I can enjoy a good TV or radio program or book:

0 ☐ Often	2 ☐ Not often
1 ☐ Sometimes	3 ☐ Hardly at all

Figure A.2.1 Hospital Anxiety and Depression Scale (continued). *A* anxiety, *D* depression. (Data from Zigmond and Snaith [1]. © 1983, reproduced with permission from John Wiley & Sons)

Distress thermometer

First: please circle the number (0–10) that best describes how much distress you have been experiencing in the past week including today

Extreme distress

10
9
8
7
6
5
4
3
2
1
0

No distress

Second: please indicate if any of the following has been a problem for you in the past week including today.
Be sure to check "Yes" or "No" for each

Practical problems

	Yes	No
Child care	☐	☐
Housing	☐	☐
Insurance/financial	☐	☐
Transportation	☐	☐
Work/school	☐	☐

Family problems

	Yes	No
Dealing with children	☐	☐
Dealing with partner	☐	☐
Dealing with close friend/relative	☐	☐

Emotional problems

	Yes	No
Depression	☐	☐
Fears	☐	☐
Nervousness	☐	☐
Sadness	☐	☐
Worry	☐	☐

	Yes	No
Loss of interest in usual activities	☐	☐
Spiritual/religious concerns	☐	☐

Physical problems

	Yes	No
Appearance	☐	☐
Bathing/dressing	☐	☐
Breathing	☐	☐
Changes in urination	☐	☐
Constipation	☐	☐
Diarrhea	☐	☐
Eating	☐	☐
Fatigue	☐	☐
Feeling swollen	☐	☐

Other problems

	Yes	No
Fevers	☐	☐
Getting around	☐	☐
Indigestion	☐	☐
Memory/concentration	☐	☐
Mouth sores	☐	☐
Nausea	☐	☐
Nose dry/congested	☐	☐
Pain	☐	☐
Sexual	☐	☐
Skin (dry/itchy)	☐	☐
Sleep	☐	☐
Tingling in hands/feet	☐	☐

Figure A.2.2 Distress thermometer. (Data from Jacobsen et al. [2]. © 2008, reproduced with permission from SAGE)

Abbreviated Mental Test Score

1. Age ☐
2. Time to nearest hour ☐
3. An address – for example 42 West Street – to be repeated by the patient at the end ☐ of the test
4. Year ☐
5. Name of hospital, residential institution or home address, depending on where ☐ the patient is situated
6. Recognition of two persons – for example, doctor, nurse, home help, etc ☐
7. Date of birth ☐
8. Year the first World War started ☐
9. Name of present monarch ☐
10. Count backwards from 20 to 1 ☐

Total score:

Each question scores one point. A score of less than six suggests dementia

Figure A.2.3 Abbreviated Mental Test Score. (Hodkinson [3]. Reproduced with permission from Oxford University Press)

Brief Pain Inventory

Date: Time:

Name: _____ _____ _____
Last First Middle initial

1. Throughout our lives, most of us have had pain from time to time (such as minor headaches, sprains, and toothaches.) Have you had pain other than these everyday kinds of pain today?

   1.☐ Yes 2.☐ No

2. On the diagram, shade in the areas where you feel pain. Put an "X" on the area that hurts the most

Figure A.2.4 Brief Pain Inventory (continued opposite).

Brief Pain Inventory

3. Please rate your pain by circling the one number that describes your pain at its *worst* in the last 24 hours

No pain | 0 1 2 3 4 5 6 7 8 9 10 | Pain as bad as you can imagine

4. Please rate your pain by circling the one number that best describes your pain at its *least* in the last 24 hours

No pain | 0 1 2 3 4 5 6 7 8 9 10 | Pain as bad as you can imagine

5. Please rate your pain by circling the one number that best describes your pain on the *average*

No pain | 0 1 2 3 4 5 6 7 8 9 10 | Pain as bad as you can imagine

6. Please rate your pain by circling the one number that tells how much pain you have *right now*

No pain | 0 1 2 3 4 5 6 7 8 9 10 | Pain as bad as you can imagine

7. What treatments or medications are you receiving for your pain?

_____

_____

8. In the last 24 hours, how much relief have pain treatments or medications provided? Please circle the one percentage that most shows how much *relief* you have received

No relief | 0% 10% 20% 30% 40% 50% 60% 70% 80% 90% 100% | Complete relief

9. Circle the one number that describes how, during the past 24 hours, pain has interfered with your:

A. Generaly activity

Does not interfere | 0 1 2 3 4 5 6 7 8 9 10 | Completely interferes

B. Mood

Does not interfere | 0 1 2 3 4 5 6 7 8 9 10 | Completely interferes

C. Walking ability

Does not interfere | 0 1 2 3 4 5 6 7 8 9 10 | Completely interferes

Figure A.2.4 Brief Pain Inventory (continued overleaf).

Brief Pain Inventory

D. Normal work (includes both work outside the home and housework)

Does not interfere   0 1 2 3 4 5 6 7 8 9 10   Completely interferes

E. Relations with other people

Does not interfere   0 1 2 3 4 5 6 7 8 9 10   Completely interferes

F. Sleep

Does not interfere   0 1 2 3 4 5 6 7 8 9 10   Completely interferes

G. Enjoyment of life

Does not interfere   0 1 2 3 4 5 6 7 8 9 10   Completely interferes

Figure A.2.4 Brief Pain Inventory (continued). (Cleeland [4] Reproduced with permission from Oxford University Press)

Leeds Assessment of Neuropathic Symptoms and Signs

Name: Date:

This pain scale can help to determine whether the nerves that are carrying your pain signals are working normally or not. It is important to find this out in case different treatments are needed to control your pain

A. Pain questionnaire

- Think about how youir pain has felt over the last week
- Please say whether any of the descriptions match your pain exactly

1. **Does your pain feel like strange, unpleasant sensations in your skin?**
   Words like pricking, tingling, pins and needles might describe these sensations

   a) No, my pain doesn't really feel like this   (0)
   b) Yes, I get these sensations quite a lot   (5)

2. **Does your pain make the skin in the painful area look different from normal?**
   Words like mottled or looking more red or pink might describe the appearance

   a) No, my pain doesn't affect the color of my skin   (0)
   b) Yes, I've noticed that the pain does make my skin look different from normal   (5)

3. **Does your pain make the affected skin abnormally sensitive to touch? Getting**
   unpleasant sensations when lightly stroking the skin, or getting pain when wearing
   tight clothes might describe the abnormal sensitivity

   a) No, my pain doesn't make my skin abnormally sensitive in the area   (0)
   b) Yes, my skin seems abnormally sensitive to touch in that area   (3)

Figure A.2.5 Leeds assessment of neuropathic symptoms and signs (continued opposite).

Leeds Assessment of Neuropathic Symptoms and Signs

4. Does your pain come on suddenly and in bursts for no apparent reason when you're still. Words like electric shocks, jumping, and bursting describe these sensations

   a) No, my pain doesn't really feel like this (0)
   b) Yes, I get these sensations quite a lot (2)

5. Does your pain feel as if the skin temperature in the painful area has change dabnormally? Words like hot and burning describe these sensations

   a) No, I don't really get these sensations (0)
   b) Yes, I get these sensations quite a lot (1)

B. Sensory testing

Skin sensitivity can be examined by comparing the painful area with a contralateral or adjacent non-painful area for the presence of allodynia and an altered pin-prick threshold (PPT)

1. Allodynia

Examine the response to lightly stroking cotton wool across the non-painful area and then the painful area. If normal sensations are experienced in the non-painful site, but pain or unpleasant sensations (tingling, nausea) are experienced in the painful area when stroking, allodynia is present

   a) No, normal sensation in both areas (0)
   b) Yes, allodynia in painful area only (5)

2. Altered pin-prick threshold

Determine the pin-prick threshold by comparing the response to a 23 gauge (blue) needle mounted inside a 2 ml syringe barrel placed gently gently on to the skin in a non-painful and then painful areas

If a sharp pin prick is felt in the non-painful area, but a different sensation is experienced in the painful area, eg, none/blunt only (raised PPT) or a very painful and then painful sensation (lowered PPT), an altered PPT is present

   a) No, equal sensation in both areas (0)
   b) Yes, altered PPT in painful area (3)

Total score
(maximum 24)

Scoring: add values in parentheses for sensory description and examination findings to obtain overall score.

If score <12, neuropathic mechanism are **unlikely** to be contributing to the patient's pain
If score ≥12, neuropathic mechanism are **likely** to be contributing to the patient's pain

Figure A.2.5 Leeds assessment of neuropathic symptoms and signs (continued). (Bennett [5]. This scale has been reproduced with permission of the International Association for the Study of Pain®. The scale may not be reproduced for any other purpose without permission)

Dermatome map of the body

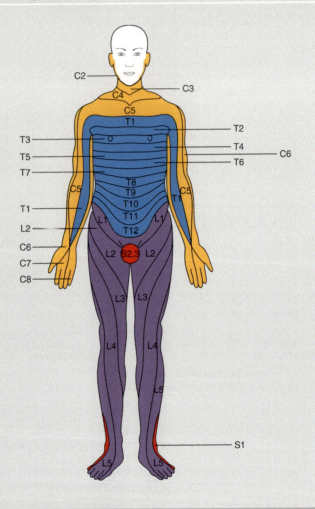

Levels of principal dermatomes

C5	Clavicles	**C8**	Ring and little fingers
C5, 6, 7	Lateral parts of upper limbs	**T4**	Level of nipples
C8, T1	Medial sides of upper limbs	**T10**	Level of umbilicus
C6	Thumb	**T12**	Inguinal or groin regions
C6, 7, 8	Hand	**L1, 2, 3, 4**	Anterior and inner surfaces of lower limbs

Figure A.2.6 Dermatome map of the body. (Reproduced with permission from Netter [6])

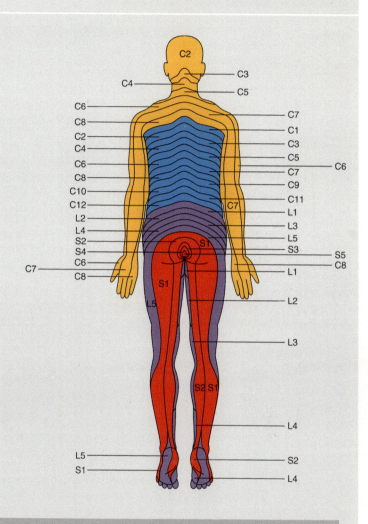

L4, 5, S1	Foot	S1	Lateral margin of foot and little toe
L4	Medial side of big toe		
S1, 2, L5	Posterior and outer surfaces of lower limbs	S2, 3, 4	Perineum

Schematic demarcation of dermatomes shown as distinct segments. There is actually considerable overlap between any two adjacent dermatomes

Breakthrough Pain Assessment Schedule

Each pain should be marked on a separate sheet

Location

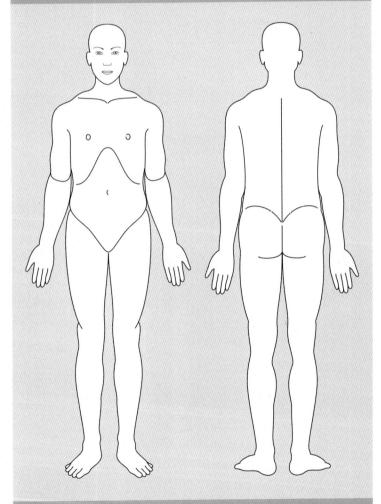

Type

A. ☐ No background pain

B. ☐ Controlled background pain

C. ☐ Uncontrolled background pain

1. ☐ No scheduled analgesia

2. ☐ Insufficient scheduled analgesia

3. ☐ Sufficient scheduled analgesia

Figure A.2.7 Breakthrough Pain Assessment Schedule (continued opposite).

Breakthrough Pain Assessment Schedule

Temporal characteristics

Daily frequency _____

Onset:

☐ Gradual

☐ Sudden

Time course:

Time to max intensity (minutes) _____

Total duration (minutes) _____

Precipitating event

☐ None (spontaneous)

☐ Incident

☐ Non-volitional

Predictable

☐ Yes

☐ No

Severity

☐ Mild

☐ Moderate

☐ Severe

☐ Excruciating

Pathophysiology

☐ Somatic

☐ Visceral

☐ Neuropathic

☐ Mixed

☐ Unknown

Etiology

☐ Disease related

☐ Treatment related

☐ Unrelated to disease/treatment

Figure A.2.7 Breakthrough Pain Assessment Schedule (continued). (Zeppetella and Ribeiro [7], reproduced with permission from SAGE publications)

Appendix 3

Formulary

The section is intended to provide a brief guide to drugs commonly used in a palliative care setting and which are mentioned in this guide:

- Figure A.3.1 Formulary.
- Figure A.3.2 Step 2 combination preparations and daily morphine equivalent.
- Figure A.3.3 Approximate hypnotics – equivalent dose of benzodiazepines.
- Figure A.3.4 Equivalent anti-inflammatory doses of corticosteroids.

For further more detailed information including contraindications, precautions, adverse effects, drug interactions, and cautions in special circumstances please see:

1. British National Formulary. Available at: www.bnf.org.
2. Dickman A. Drugs in palliative care. Oxford: Oxford University Press; 2010.
3. Twycross R, Wilcox A, editors. Palliative care formulary. 3rd edn. Available at: www.palliativedrugs.com.

Formulary (continued)

Drug	Preparation	Indications	Dose
Alfentanil	Injection: 500 µg/mL (2 and 10 mL) 5 mg/mL (1 mL)	Opioid for moderate-to-severe pain often administered by CSCI	Requires titration Typical starting dose 250-500 µg sc prn or 1mg/24 h CSCI
Amitriptyline	Tablets: 10, 25, 50 mg Liquid: 25 or 50 mg/5 mL	Depression Neuropathic pain Bladder spasm	Depression 75-100 mg/day Neuropathic pain start at 10-25 mg, titrate to75 mg
Anastrazole	Tablets: 1 mg	Breast cancer in post-menopausal women	1mg/day
Baclofen	Tablets: 10 mg Liquid: 5 mg/5 mL	Spasticity Hiccup	Titrate from 5–10 mg/day to 100 mg/day
Bethanecol	Tablets: 10 mg 25 mg	Dry mouth	10–25 mg tds
Bisocodyl	Tablets: 5 mg Suppository:10 mg	Constipation	Oral:5–20 mg od/bd Rectally: 10 mg prn
Benzydamine	Oral rinse: 0.15%	Painful inflammation of oropharynx	4–8 sprays on to affected area every 1.5–3 h
Buprenorphine	Transdermal BuTrans patch, 5, 10, or 20 µg/ hour for 7 days Transdermal Transtec patch: 35, 52.5, or 70 µg/hour over 4 days	Moderate-to-severe pain	Titrate through dose range
Capsaicin	0.025% or 0.075% cream	Neuropathic pain	Apply sparingly up to tds/qds (not more often than every 4h)
Capsaicin (TD)	Self-adhesive patch containing capsaicin 8%	Peripheral neuropathic pain in non-diabetic patients to a maximum of 4 patches	Should be applied to the most painful skin areas

Figure A.3.1 Formulary (continued overleaf).

Notes

A synthetic fentanyl derivative with a more rapid onset of action, a shorter duration of action, and a potency approximately 25% that of fentanyl
Usually reserved for patients unable to tolerate morphine or diamorphine
(eg, renal failure) 1mg alfentanil ≡ 10 mg diamorphine

Blocks the presynaptic reuptake of serotonin and norepinephrine
Adjuvant analgesic for neuropathic pain
Analgesic effect usually seen at lower doses and more quickly than antidepressant effect; anticholinergic adverse effects may be troublesome

Adjuvant treatment of estrogen receptor-positive, early, invasive breast cancer in post-menopausal women; adjuvant treatment of estrogen receptor-positive, early breast cancer inpost-menopausal women after 2–3 years of tamoxifen therapy; advanced breast cancer in post-menopausal women that is estrogen receptor positive or responsive to tamoxifen

Acts on the GABA receptor, inhibiting the release of the excitatory amino acids glutamate and aspartate, thereby decreasing spasm in skeletal muscle

Spasticity: increase dose slowly to usual daily max of 100 mg
Can be delivered by implantable spinal pump
Baclofen relieves hiccup, possibly by a direct effect on the diaphragm

Adverse effects include nausea, vomiting, diarrhea, abdominal pain, flushing, hypotension, headache, and sweating

Stimulant laxative to be avoided in complete bowel obstruction
Oral formulation works within 12 h, rectal formulation within 1 h
Avoid in bowel obstruction

Adverse effects can include numbness or stinging, in which case can be diluted with water

Buprenorphine is highly lipid soluble, making it suitable for transdermal delivery
Usual max dose is 140 µg/hour. Appears to acts as full agonist in therapeutic range; other opioids can be used for breakthrough pain
Sublingual table available (Temgesic 200 or 400 µg)
Injection : 300 µg/mL

Affects the synthesis, storage, transport, and release of substance P in pain fibers
Start with lowest strength and wear gloves to administer

A self-adhesive patch containing capsaicin 8% is licensed for the treatment of peripheral neuropathic pain in non-diabetic patients

Applied to intact skin, for 30 – 60 min, depending on cause of pain; can be repeated every 90 days

Formulary (continued)

Drug	Preparations	Indications	Dose
Carbamazepine	Tablet: 100, 200, or 400 mg Liquid: 100 mg/5 mL Suppository: 125 or 250 mg	Generalized and partial seizures Neuropathic pain	Titrate starting with 100–200 mg/day and increase by 100–200 mg every 2 weeks. Usual response range 400–600 mg bd
Carbocisteine	Capsule: 375 mg Liquid: 125 or 250 mg/5mL	Reduces sputum viscosity and aids expectoration	Start 750 mg tds
Celecoxib	Capsule: 100 or 200 mg	Pain	Initial dose 100 mg bd and increase to 200 mg bd if required
Citalopram	Tablet: 10, 20, or 40 mg Oral drops: 40 mg/mL	Depression Panic Pain	Depression: 20 mg od increased if necessary to max 60 mg/day Panic or pain: initially 10 mg/day increased to 20–30 mg/day; max 60 mg/day
Clonazepam	Tablet: 0.5 or 2 mg Injection: 1 mg/mL	Epilepsy Myoclonus Neuropathic pani Terminal restlessness	1 mg initially on for 4 nights, increased over 2–4 weeks to usual maintenance dose of 4–8 mg usually at night CSCI 1–4 mg/24 h
Co-danthramer	Capsule: 25/200 or 37.5/500 (strong) Suspension: 25/200 in 5 mL or 75/1000 (strong) in 5 mL	Constipation in terminally ill patients	Capsule: 1 or 2 od and then titrate Supension: 5–10 mL od and then titrate Increase to 'strong' as necessary
Codeine	Tablet: 15, 30 or 60 mg syrup: 25 mg/5mL Linctus: 15 mg/mL Injection: 60 mg/mL	Mild/moderate pain Diarrhea Cough	Pain: 30–60 mg every 4 h Max daily close: 240 mg Diarrhea: 30 mg qds Cough: 5–10 mL (linctus) qds

Figure A.3.1 Formulary (continued overleaf).

Notes

Adjuvant analgesic for neuropathic pain

Titrate slowly by 100–200 mg every 2 weeks, usual max daily close 800–1200 mg in divided closes, occasionally 1.6–2.0 g

Standard and modified-release preparations available

Watch for drug interactions and blood dyscrasias

Reduce dose to 750 mg bd once satisfactory response obtained

Discontinue after 2 weeks if no response

For depression increase at intervals of 3–4 weeks in steps of 20 mg; people age > 65 years, max 40 mg/day
For panic increase gradually in steps of 10 mg; People age > 65 years, max 40 mg/day

In people age > 65 years start with 500 μg

Increase according to response over 2–4 weeks

Max close may be given in three to four divided closes if necessary

Combination of stimulant and softener

Co-danthramer suspension 5 mL ≡ 1 co-danthramer capsule

Strong co-danthramer suspension 5 mL ≡ strong co-danthramer capsules
Warn patients that urine may be colored red or orange
Prolonged contact with skin can causes 'co-danthramer burn'

One-tenth potency of morphine

Some white people are poor metabolizers of codeine; other ethnic groups may be extensive or ultra-metabolizers

Combination products available (see Figure 6.7)

Formulary (continued)

Drug	Preparations	Indications	Dose
Cyclizine	Tablet: 50 mg Injection: 50 mg/mL	Nausea Vomiting	50–100 mg po or sc 100–150 mg/24 h via CSCI Max daily oral/ subcutaneous dose: 200 mg
Cyproterone	Tablet: 50 or 100 mg	Prostate cancer	200–300 mg/day in two to three divided doses
Dexamethasone	Tablet: 0.5 or 2 mg Oral solution: 2 mg/5 mL Injection: 8 mg/2 mL or 4 mg/mL	Cerebral edema Anorexia Dyspnea Nausea Vomiting Pain SCC SVCO	Daily dose ranges from 2 to 16 mg depending indication
Diamorphine	Tablet: 10 mg Injection: 5, 10, 30, 100, or 500 mg	Pain Breathlessness	Requires titration CSCI: typical starting dose 10–20 mg/24 h
Diazepam	Tablet: 2, 5, or 10 mg Oral solution: 2 mg/5 mL or 5 mg/mL Injection: 5 mg/mL Rectal solution: 2.5 mg/1.25 mL, 5 mg/2.5 mL, or 10 mg/5 mL Suppository: 10 mg	Anxiety Insomnia Myoclonus Seizures	Initial dose 2 mg and titrate depending on effect for each indication
Diclofenac	Tablet: 25 or 50 mg Dispersible tablet 50 mng injection: 75 mg Suppository: 12.5, 25, 50, or 100 mg	Pain Inflammation	Orally or rectally: 75–150 mg/day in divided doses
Diethylstilbestrol	Tablet: 1 mg	Prostate cancer	Initially 1 mg/day Can be increased to 3 mg

Figure A.3.1 Formulary (continued overleaf).

Notes

Useful for vomiting due to gastrointestinal causes or raised intracranial pressure
Subcutaneous route may cause skin reactions
Can precipitate with Buscopan if both given in syringe driver

Can be used to treat flare with intial gonadorlin therapy (300 mg/day bd/tds, reduced
to 200 mg/day bd/tds if necessary) or hot flushes with gonadorelin therapy or
after orchidectomy intially 50 mg/day, adjusted according to
response to 50–150 mg/day od/tds

Appetite and fatigue 2–4 mg
Nerve compression, vomiting, breathlessness: 8–12 mg
SCC, SCVO, raised intracranial pressure: 16 mg (sometimes higher)
Metabolism accelerated by carbamazepine and phenytoin (reduced effect)
Doses best given in the morning
Can be delivered by CSCI
Consider PPI if risk of peptic ulceration
Remember to give patient a steroid card

Often preferred for injection because, being more soluble, it can be given in a
smaller volume
Reduce dose in elderly people and patients with renal failure

Benzodiazepine with GABA-potentiating actions in the CNS
Long plasma half-life and several active metabolites
Anxiety: 2–10 mg po, usual range 2–20 mg po
Muscle spasm: 2–5 mg po, usual range 2–20 mg po
Anticonvulsant: 10 mg pr/iv, usual range 10–30 mg
Rectal solutions available

Consider PPI if risk of peptic ulceration
Available with misoprostol (Arthrotec 50 or 75) and as a modified-release
preparation: 75 and 100 mg.

Under specialist supervision
Also used (uncommonly) for breast cancer in post-menopausal women

Formulary (continued)

Drug	Preparations	Indications	Dose
Dihydrocodeine	Tablet: 30 or 40 (Forte mg Oral Soultion 10 mg/5 mL Injection: 50 mg/mL)	Moderate/sever pain	30–60 mg every 4 h Max daily dose: 240 mg
Docusate sodium	Capsule: 100 mg Oral solution 12.5 or 50 mg/5 mL enema: 120 mg in 10 g	Constipation Partial bowel obstruction	Orally: 100 mg bd and titrated to max dose 200 mg tds
Domperidone	Tablet: 10 mg Suspension: 5 mg/5mL Suppository: 30 mg	Nausea Vomiting Gastroesophageal reflux Dyspepsia	Orally: 10–20 mg tds/qds Max daily dose 80 mg Rectally: 60 mg bd
Etamsylate	Tablet: 500 mg	Capillary bleeding	Orally: 500 mg qds
Fentanyl	Transdermal patches: 12, 25, 50, 75, or 100 µg/hour Transmucosal systems Buccal lozenge (Actiq): 200, 400, 600, 800, 1200, or 1600 µg Sublingual tablet (Abstral): 100, 200, 300, 400, 600, or 800 µg Buccal tablet (Effentora): 100, 200, 400, 600, or 800 µg Nasal spray (Instanyl): 50,100, or 200 µg per spray Nasal spray (PecFent): 100 or 400 µg per spray	Transdermal patches: moderate-to-severe cancer pain Buccal lozenge, sublingual tablet, buccal tablet, and nasal sprays: Breakthrough cancer pain	Transdermal systems Requires titration Transmucosal systems Requires titration
Fluconanzole	Capsule: 50, 150, or 200 mg Suspension: 50 mg/5 mL or 200 mg/mL	Mucosal candidiasis Genital candidiasis	Mucosal candidiasis: 50 mg od 100 mg od in resistant cases Genital candidiasis: 150 mg po as single dose

Figure A.3.1 Formulary (continued overleaf).

Notes

Modified-release preparations available (DHC Continus 60, 90 or 12
Combination products available (see Figure A3.2)

Soften stools and is weak stimulant
Acts in 1–2 days
Do not give with liquid paraffin
Rectal preparations not indicated if hemorrhoids or anal fissure

Can sometimes cause gastrointestinal disturbances (including cramps)
Fewer extrapyramidal problems than metoclopramide

Reduces capillary bleeding in the presence of a normal number of platelets. It does
not act by fibrin stabilization, but probably by correcting abnormal adhesion
Can cause nausea, headache, or rashes

Fentanyl patch preparations include the matrix systems Durogesic DTrans,
Matrifen, and Mezolar, and the reservoir system Fentalis. It is not
possible to ensure interchangeability of the different formulations

Transmucosal opioids are licensed for breakthrough cancer pain in
patients on background opioid maintenance therapy. It is not possible to
ensure interchangeability of the different formulations, hence if switching
retitration is recommended

Cautions with concomitant use with hepatotoxic drugs, monitor liver function
with high doses or extended courses – discontinue if signs or symptoms of hepatic
disease (risk of hepatic necrosis); susceptibility to QT interval prolongation
Can cause nausea, abdominal discomfort, diarrhea, flatulence, headache, rash
(discontinue treatment or monitor closely if infection invasive or systemic)

Formulary (continued)

Drug	Preparations	indications	Dose
Fluoxetine	Capsule: 20 mg Liquid: 20 mg/ 5 mL	Depression Anxiety	Initial dose 20 mg Max dose 60 mg /day
Flutamide	Tablet: 250 mg	Prostate cancer	250 mg tds
Furosemide	Tablet: 20, 40, or 500 mg Oral solution: 20, 40, or 50 mg/5 mL Injection; 20 mg/2 mL, 50 mg/5 mL, or 250 mg/25 mL	Edema	40 Mg od In resistant cases 80–120 mg/day
Gabapentin	Capsule: 100, 300, or 400 mg Tablet: 600 or 800 mg	Neuropathic pain\ Seizures Restless leg syndrome	Initial dose 300 mg Increasing gradually to a max dose 3.6 mg
Glycopyrronium	Injection: 200 µg/mL	Excessive secretions	Orally: 0.6–1 mg tds Subcutaneously: 0.2 –0.4 mg CSCI: 0.6–1.2 mg/24 h
Haloperidol	Capsule: 500 µg Tablet: 0.5, 1.5, 5, 10, or 20 mg Oral solution: 1 or 2 mg/mL Injection: 5 mg/mL	Psychosis Hiccup Restlessness Agitation Delirium Nausea Vomiting	Antiemetic: initial dose 1.5 mg/day Antipsychotic: initial dose 5 mg/day Intractable hiccup: Initial dose 1.5 mg/day
Hydromorphone	Capsule: 1.3 or 2.6 mg Injection: 10, 20, or 50 mg/mL	Severe cancer pain	requires titration
Hyoscine Butylbromide (Scopolamine butylbromide)	Tablet: 10 mg Injection: 20 mg /mL	Smooth muscle spasm Nausea Vomiting Excessive secretions Sweating	Smooth muscle colic:start with 20 mg sc start and 60 mg/24 h CSCI Secretions: start with 20 mg sc stat, 20–60 mg/24 h CSCI

Figure A.3.1 Formulary (continued overleaf).

Notes

Dose can be gradually increased from initial dose after 3–4 weeks

Adverse effects include gynecomastia (sometimes with galactorrhea); nausea, vomiting, diarrhea, increased appetite, insomnia, and tiredness

Usually acts within 1 h of oral administration and diuresis is complete within 6 h so that, if necessary, they can be given twice a day without interfering with sleep Should be avoided in severe hypokalemia, severe hyponatremia

In normal renal function: 300 mg od on day 1, then 300 mg bd on day 2, then 300 mg tds on day 3, or initially 300 mg tds on day 1, then increased according to response in steps of 300mg tds every 2–3 days up to max 3.6 g/day
Slower titration over several weeks is advisable in debilitated and elderly patients, those with renal impairment, or if receiving other CNS depressent drugs: 100 mg tds onday 1, then 300 mg tds on day 7, then 600 mg tds day 14, incresase by 300 mg/day every 3 days as needed upto 1200 mg tds

Occasionally doses of up to 2 mg tds are needed
Can cause inflammation at the injection site
An oral solution 1 mg/10 mL (0.01%) can be prepared extemporaneously for individual patients from glycopyrronium powder

Antiemetic: intial dose 1.5 mg/day stat asnd typical maintenance dose 1.5–3 mg/day; if necessary, increased dose progressively to 5–10 mg/day
Antipsychotic: intial dose 5 mg stat (1.5 mg in elderly people) and, if necessary, increase daily dose progresssively to 20–30 mg in divided doses. if the patient does not settle with 20 mg/day, consider prescribing a benzodiazepine concurrently
Intractable hiccup: maintenance dose 1.5–3 mg/day

Modified-release preparation available (Palladone SR 2, 4, 8,16, and 24 mg)

Smooth muscle colic: start with 20 mg sc start and 60 mg/24 CSCI and, if necessary increase to 120 mg/24 h, max dose 300 mg /24 h
Some center add octreotide 300–500 μg/24 h if hyoscine (scopolamine) buty bromide 120 mg/24 h fails to relieve symptoms adequately
For patients with obstructive symptoms without colic, metoclopramide should be tried before an antimuscarinic drug because the obstruction is often more functional than organic
Secretions: start with 20 mg sc stat, 20–60 mg/24 h CSCI, and 20 mg sc q 1h prn. Some centers use higher doses, namely 60–120 mg/24 h CSCI

Formulary

Drug	Preparations	Indications	Dose
Hyoscine hydrobromide (scopolamine hydrobromide)	Tablet: 150 or 300 µg TD patch: 1.5 mg Injection: 400 or 600 µg	Motion sickness Drooling Smooth muscle spasm Nausea Vomiting Excessive secretions Sweating	Drooling: transdermal hyoscine hydrobromide 1 mg/72 h Secretions: 400 ug sc stat
Ibuprofen	Tablet: 200, 400, or 600 mg Effervescent granules: 600 mg Syrup: 100 mg/5 mL Oral suspension: 100 mg/5 mL	Mild/moderate pain	Initial dose 300–400 mg tds/qds
Ketamine	Injection: 10, 50, or 100 mg/mL	Pain unresponsive to standard therapies	Orally: initial dose 10–25 mg tds/qds Sublingually: start with 10–25 mg Subcutaneously: typically 10–25 mg prn CSCI: start with 1–2.5 mg/kg per 24 h
Lactulose	Solution: 3.1–3.7 g/5 mL	Constipation Hepatic encephalopathy	15 mL bd
Lansoprazole	Capsule: 15 or 30 mg Orodispersible tablet: 15 or 30 mg		15–30 mg od
Levomepromazine	Tablet: 6 or 25 mg Injection: 25 mg/mL	Psychosis Nausea Vomiting Terminal agitation	Orally: 3 mg od/bd Subcutaneously: 6–12.5 mg CSCIP: 12.5–75 mg

Figure A.3.1 Formulary (continued overleaf).

Notes

Secretions: initial dose 400 μg sc stat and then continue with 1200 μg/24 h
CSCI, if necessary increase to 2000 μg/ 24 h CSCI repeat 400 μg prn
Some centers use hyoscine (scopolamine) butylbromide instead. It is cheaper than
hyoscine (scopolamine) hydrobromide
Other options include glycopyrronium

Can be increased if necessary to max 2.4 g/day; maintenance dose of
0.6–1.2 g/day may be adequate
Modified–release preparation available (Brufen Retard 800 mg,
Fenbid Spansule 300 mg)

Orally: if necessary, increase dose in steps of 10–25 mg up to 50 mg qds; max
reported dose 200 mg qds. Oral solution (50 mg/mL is available as an
unlicensed special
Subcutaneously: some use 2.5–5 mg if necessary, increase dose in steps of 25–33%
CSCI: if necessary, increase by 50–100 mg/24 h, max reported dose 3.6 g/24 h
Alternatively, give as short-term "burst" therapy: start with 100 mg/ 24 h,
and increase if required to 300 mg/24 h on day 2 and 500 mg/24 h on
day 3. Stop 3 days after last dose increment

May take up to 48 h to act
Adverse effects include abdominal bloating, flatulence, nausea, and intestinal colic
In hepatic encephalopathy dose: 30–50 mL po tds

Benign gastric ulcer: 30 mg/day in the morning for 8 weeks
Duodenal ulcer: 30 mg/day in the morning for 4 weeks; maintenance 15 mg/day
NSAID- associated duodenal or gastric ulcer: 30 mg od for 4 weeks,
Continued for further 4 weeks if not fully healed
NSAID-associated duodenal or gastric ulcer prophylaxis, 15–30 mg od
Gastroesophageal reflux disease: 30 mg/day in the morning for 4 weeks,
continued for further 4 weeks if not fully healed; maintenance 15–30 mg/day
Acid-related dyspepsia, 15–30 mg/day in the morning for 2–4 weeks

First-line antiemetic, start with 3 mg od/bd and, if necessary, increase to 6 mg od/bd
Second-line antimetic starting with 6–12.5 mg po/sc stat and, if necessary,
increaseing top 25–50 mg/24 h
Terminal agitation or delirium: starting dose 25 mg sc and 50–75 mg/24 h CSCI
titrated according to reponse; max 300 mg /24 h, occasionally more

Formulary (continued)

Drug	Preparations	Indications	Dose
Lidocaine	Ointment: lidocaine hydrochloride 5% Solution: lidocaine hydrochloride 4% Medicated plaster: 5% w/w lidocaine (700 mg)	Topical analgesia PHN	Topical analgesia: 1–2 mL applied when necessary PHN: 1–3 patches for 12 h a day
Loperamide	Capsule: 2 mg Tablet: 2 mg syrup: 1 mg/5 mL	Acute diarrhea Chronic diarrhea Fecal incontinence	2–4 mg stat
Lorazepam	Tablet: 1 or 2.5 mg Injection: 4 mg/mL	Seizures Insomnia Anxiety Agitation	1–4 mg od/bd
Macrogol "3350"	Oral powder: 6.563 or 13.125 g Macrogol "3350"	Constipation Fecal impaction	Chronic constipation one to three sachets/day, Fecal impaction: eight sachets/day
Medroxyprogesterone	Tablet: 100, 200, or 400 mg	Endometrial cancer Breast cancer in post-menopausal women Anorexia	400 mg od/bd
Megesterol	Tablet: 160 mg	Endometrial cancer Breast cancer in post-menopausal women Anorexia	40–160 mg od
Methadone	Tablet: 5 mg Oral solution: 1, 5, 10, or 20 mg/mL Linctus: 2 mg/5 mL Injection: 1 mg/mL	Moderate/severe pain	Titrated

Figure A.3.1 Formulary (continued overleaf).

Notes

PHN: apply plaster to intact, dry non-irritated skin od for up to 12 h, followed by a 12-hour plaster-free period; discontinue if no response after 4 weeks.
Up to three plasters may be used to cover large areas; plasters may be cut

Acute diarrhea, 4 mg initially followed by 2 mg after each losse stool for up to 5 days; usual dose 6–8 mg/day; max 16 mg/day
Chronic diarrhea: intially, 4–8 mg/day in divided doses, subseauently adjusted accordings to response and given in 2 divided doses for maintenance; max 16 mg/day
Fecal incontinence (unlicensed indication, intially 500 µg/day adjusted to reponse; max 16 mg/day in divided doses

Insomnia: 2-4 mg po
Anxiety: 1 mg sl/po stat bd; if necessary, increase to 2–6 mg/24 h
Acute psychotic agitation: 2 mg po/30 minutes until the patient is settled, often used with haloperidol or risperidone to control psychotic agitation

Inert polymers of ethylene glycol, which sequester fluid in the bowel
Chronic constipation, one to three sachets daily in divided doses usually for up to 2 weeks; contents of each sachet dissolved in half a glass (approximately 125 mL) of water; maintenance, one to two sachets/day
Fecal impaction: eight sachets/day dissolved in 1L of water and drunk within 6 h, usually for max 3 days

Takes 2–3 weeks to produce a maximal effect

Takes 2–3 weeks to produce a maximal effect

Long half-life
Can be used in renal failure
Caution if switching from another opioid as conversion factor highly variable and often dose dependent. Switching is best done with specialist support and if possible as an inpatient

Formulary (continued)

Drug	Preparations	Indications	Dose
Methynaltrexone	Injection: 12 mg/0.6mL, 20 mg/mL	Constipation	Initial dose 8 mg (patients weighing 38–61 Kg) or 12 mg (patients weighing 62–114 kg)
Metoclopramide	Tablet: 10 mg Syrup: 5 mg/5 mL Injection: 10 mg/2 mL	Nausea Vomiting Dyspepsia Reflex	Orally: 10–20 mg qds CSCI: 30–100 mg/24 h
Metronidazole	Gel: 0.75% Tablet: 200 or 400 mg Oral suspension: 200 mg/5 mL Suppository: 500 mg Injection: 100 mg/20 mL 500 mg/100 mL	Anerobic infections	400–800 mg tds
Midazolam	Injection: 2 mg/2 mL, 5 mg/ 5 mL, 50 mg/50 mL 10 mg/5 mL 10 mg/2 mL, or 50 mg/10 mL	Myoclonus Seizures Terminal agitation Intractable hiccup Nausea Vomiting	Subcutaneous: 5 mg stat and prn doses
Mirtazepine	Tablet: 15, 30, or 45 mg Orodispersible tablet: 15, 30, or 45 mg Oral solution: 15 mg/mL	Depression Anorexia Nausea Vomiting Pruritus	Initially 15–30 mg in the evening
Modafinil	Tablet: 100 or 200 mg	Cancer-related fatigue	200 mg od

Figure A.3.1 Formulary (continued overleaf).

Notes

Initially give a single dose on alternate days. If there is no response, a second dose can be given after 24 h, but not more often. Alternatively the interval can be extended. Approximately 50% patients defecate within 4 h of a dose with out impairment of analgesia or the development of withdrawal symptoms

Common undesirable effects include abdominal pain, diarrhea, flatulence, and nausea In severe reenal impairment (creatinie clearance < 30 mL/min), the dose should be reduced. It is contraindicated in the presence of known or suspected GI obstruction

Gastric irritation: 10 mg po qds or 40–60 mg/24 h CSCI; prescribe gastroprotective drug

Delayed gastric emptying: 10 mg po qds or 40–100 mg/ 24 h CSCI

Nausea and vomiting: 10–20 mg qds. Increases gastric motlilty and gastric emptying

Use cautiously in GI obstruction

Modified-release preparation available (Maxolon SR 15 mg)

Anerobic infections (usually treated for 7 days and for 10–14 days in *Clostridium difficile* Infection), orally, either 800 mg initially then 400 mg tds or 500 mg tds

Myoclonus: 10–30 mg CSCI

Seizures: 30–60 mg CSCI

Terminal agitation: 30–60 mg CSCI. if the patient does not settle on 30 mg/24 h, an antipsychotic (eg, haloperidol) is best introduced before further increasing the dose of midazolam

Hiccup: 30–60 mg CSCI

Nausea/Vomiting: 10–20 mg/24 h CSCI

Midazolam can be given buccally (unlicensed route). A buccal liquid is available as an unlicensed special order, or the contents of an ampoule for injection can be used

Increased within 2–4 weeks according to reponse; max 45 mg/day od/bd

If no reponse after 4 weeks on 45 mg, switch to an alternative antidepressant.

If effective, continue until the patient has been symptom free for 6 months; then discontinue over 2–4 weeks

Reduce dose in elderly people, or those with hepatic or renal impairment

An effect should be seen within a few h of the first dose

Formulary (continued)

Drug	Preparations	Indications	Dose
Morphine	Oral solution: 10 mg/mL or 10 ng/mL Tablet: 10, 20, or 50 mg Suppository: 10, 15, 20, or 30 mg Injection: 10, 15, or 30 mg/mL	Moderate/severe pain Breathlessness Cough Diarrhea	Titrate dose Usual starting dose 5–10 mg/q4th
Naloxone	Injection: 400 µg/mL or 2 mg/2 mL	Opioid-induced respiratory depression	Intravenous: 0.4–2 mg
Naproxen	Tablet: 250 or 500 mg Tablet (EC): (250, 375, or 500 mg	Pain Inflammation	Orally: 0.5–1 g/day in one to two divided doses
Nifedipine	Capsule: 5 or 10 mg	Smooth muscle spasm Hiccup	10 mg po/sl stat and 10–20 mg tds
Nystatin	Oral suspension: 100,000 units/mL	Oral or esophageal candidiasis	1–5 mL qds held in the mouth for 1 minute, and then swallowed
Octreotide	Injection: 50 µg/mL, 100 µg/mL 1 mg/5 mL, or 500 µg/mL	Vomiting Diarrhea Bronchorrhea Ascites Rectal discharge	Intestinal obstruction: 250–500 µg/day Ascites: 200–600 µg/day Bronchorrhea: 300–500 µg/day Intractable diarrhea: 50–500 µg/day
Olanzapine	Tablet: 2.5, 5, 7.5, 10, 15, or 20 mg Orodispersible tablet: 5, 10, 15, or 20 mg Injection: 10 mg	Psychosis Nausea Vomiting Delirium Terminal agitation	Agitation: 2.5 mg stat Delirium: 2.5 mg stat Antiemetic: 1.25–2.5 mg

Figure A.3.1 Formulary (continued overleaf).

Notes

Modified-release preparations available:
Morphigesic (12-hour duration): 10, 30, 60, or 100 mg
MST Continus (12-hour duration): 5, 10, 30, 60, 100, or 200 mg
Zomorph (12-hour duration): 10, 30, 60,100 or 200 mg
MXL (24-hour duration) : 30, 60, 90,120,150, or 200 mg
Reduce dose in elderly people and patients with renal impairment

If no response repeat at intervals of 2–3 minutes to a max of 10 mg
Beware return of severe pain

Formulation with misoprostol (Napratec: naproxen 500 mg + misoprostol 200 µg)

Usual max dose 60–80 mg/day
Modified-release formulations available (10, 20, 30, or 60 mg)
Up to 160 mg/day has been used for Intractable hiccup with concurrent
fludrocortisone 0.5–1.0 mg to overcome associated orthostatic hypotension

Dentures should be removed before each dose, and clean before re-insertion
The use of locally prepared nystain popsicises is sometimes helpful; 5 mL
nystatin suspension is mixed with blackcurrant or other fruit juice concentrate
and frozen in an ice tray with small rounded cups

Intestinal obstruction: increasing to a max 750 µg/day, occasionally higher
Intestinal diarrhea: increasing to a max 1500 µg/day, occasionally higher
Once improvement in the symptom is achieved, reduction to the lowest dose
that maintains symptom control can be tried
A depot formulation of octreotide 10–30 mg, given every 4 weeks, is available and
may be of use in patients with a chronic intestinal fistula or intractable diarrhea

Agitation and/or delirium: increase if necessary to 5–10 mg od
Antiemertic: starting dose increase if necessary to 5 mg od
The higher dose may be necessary in patients receiving highly emetogenic
chemotherapy, eg, cisplatin
Orodispersible tablets are placed on the tongue and allowed to dissolve or dispersed
in water, orange juice, apple juice, milk, or coffee immediately before administration

Formulary (continued)

Drug	Preparationas	Indications	Dose
Ondansetron	Tablet: 4 or 8 mg Syrup:4 mg/5 mL Oral lyophilisate: 4 or 8 mg Injection: 4 mg/2 mL, 4 mg/5 mL, 8 mg/2 mL, or 8 mg/4 mL Suppository: 16 mg	Nausea Vomiting Pruritus	Orally: 8 mg bd/tds Subcutaneously: 8 mg bd/tds Rectally: 16 mg/day CSCI: 8-24 mg/day Pruritus: 4–8 mg bd/tds
Oxybutynin	Tablet: 2.5, 3, or 5 mg Elixir: 2.5 mg/5 mL	Urinary incontinence Urinary frequency	Initial dose 5 mg po bd increased as necessary to 5 mg po qds
Oxycodone	Oral solution: 5 mg/5 mL or 10 mg/mL Tablet: 5, 10, or 20 mg Injection: 10 mg/mL, 20 mg/2 mL, or 50 mg/mL	Moderate/severe pain Breathlessness	Titrate dose Usual starting dose 2.5–5 mg q4h
Pamidronate sodium	Injection: 15, 30, or 90 mg	Hypercalcemia Bone pain	Dependent on serum calcium: up to 3 mmol/L 15–30 mg, 3–3.5 mmol/L 30–60 mg, 3.5–4 mmol/L 60–90 mg, and >4 mmol/L 90 mg
Paracetamol	Tablet: 500 mg Caplet: 500 mg Soluble tablet: 500 mg Oral suspension: 250 mg/5 mL or 500 mg/5 mL Suppository: 60, 125, 250, or 500 mg	Mild/moderate pain Fever	Orally or rectally: 0.5–1 g q4–6h Intravenously: 1 9 q4–6h
Paroxetine	Tablet: 10, 20, and 30 mg Oral suspension: 10 mg/5 mL	Anxiety Depression Panic Pruritus	Anxiety: 20 mg in the morning Panic: 10 mg in the morning Pruritus: 5 mg in the morning

Figure A.3.1 Formulary (continued overleaf).

Notes

If a 5HT3 -receptor antagonist is not clearly effective within 3 days, it should be discontinued

If clearly of benefit, continue indefinitely unless the cause is self-limiting

Modified-release formulations available (Lyrinel XL 5 or 10 mg, Kentera transdermal patch 3.9/24 h applied for 72–96 h)

Modified-release preparations available:

Oxycontin (12-hour duration): 5, 10, 20, 40, or 80 mg

Naloxone combination preparation:

5 mg/2.5 mg oxycodone/naloxone or 10 mg/5 mg, 20 mg/10 mg, and 40 mg/20 mg

Inhibitor of osteoclastic bone resorption

Max response should be seen within 3–7 days

Osteonecrosis of the jaw a potential complication

Max dose 4 g in 24 h

Anxiety: increase gradually up to a max of 50 mg in 10-mg increments according to response

Panic: usual max of 40 mg in 10-mg increments; some patients require 60 mg

Pruritus: increase to max of 20 mg

Formulary (continued)

Drug	Preparations	Indications	Dose
Phenobarbital	Tablet: 15, 30, or 60 mg Elixir: 15 mg/5 mL Injection: 200 mg/mL	Seizures Terminal agitation	Seizures: 60–180 mg po in the morning or 200–400 mg via CSCI over 24 h Terminal agitation: initial dose 100–200 mg im or iv
Prednisolone	Tablet: 1, 5, or 25 mg Tablet (EC): 2.5 or 5 mg Tablet (soluble): 5 mg	Anorexia Suppression of inflammation	10–20 mg po od
Pregabalin	Capsule: 25, 50, 75, 100, 150, 200, 225, or 300 mg	Neuropathic pain Partial seizures Anxiety	Initial dose range 25 mg od to 75 mg bd
Propantheline	Tablet: 15 mg	Smooth muscle spasm Sweating Urinary frequency	15 mg po bd/tds
Quinine sulfate	Tablet: 200 or 300 mg	Nocurnal leg Cramps	200–300 mg in the evening
Risperidone	Tablet: 0.5, 1, 2, 3, 4, or 6 mg Orodispersible tablet: 0.5, 1, 2, 3 or 4 mg Liquid: 1 mg/mL	Psychosis Delirium Nausea Vomiting	Psychosis: 1 mg bd Delirium: 0.5 mg bd Nausea: 0.5 mg in the evening Vomiting: 0.5 mg in the evening
Senna	Tablet: 7.5 mg Syrup: 7.5 mg/5 mL	Constipation	Orally: 7.5–15 mg in the evening
Sertraline	Tablet: 50 or 100 mg	Depression Anxiety Cholestatic pruritus	50 mg od
Spironolactone	Tablet: 25, 50, or 100 mg	Ascites	100 mg od in the morning

Figure A.3.1 Formulary (continued overleaf).

Notes

Terminal agitation: continue treatment with 200–600 mg via CSCI over 24 h
Water for injection used in CSCI
Dilute in 10 times own volume; higher doses will necessitate 12-hour infusion

Dose preferably given in the morning
Dose can be reduced after a few days
Some chronic conditions require a maintenance dose 2.5–15 mg
Remember steroid card

In normal renal function: 75 mg bd on day 1,150 mg bd daily 3–7, then 300 mg bd days 10–14, then increased according to reponse to max dose of 600 mg/day
OR
25 mg on day 1, 25 mg bd day 2, 75 mg bd days 6–7, then increase by 25 mg bd every 2 days as needed to a max 600 mg/day

Increase to a max of 30 mg qds

Take dose with food to avoid GI irritation

Psychosis: increase on day 2 to 2 mg bd and can be further increased to 3 mg bd or higher, usually under expert supervision
Delirium: increase by 0.5 mg/day to a max dose 1 mg bd
Nausea/vomiting: usually max dose 1 mg in the evening

Higher doses frequently used by patients on opioids. Max dose 30 mg in the evening but up to 60 mg reported
Often used in combination with a stool softener
Stimulant laxatives increase intestinal motility and often cause abdominal cramp; they should be avoided in intestinal obstruction

Depression/anxiety: increase if necessary by 50 mg/week to 200 mg; usual maintenance is 50 mg/day
Cholestatic pruritus: dose can be increased as necessary after 7 days; usual maintenance dose is 75–100 mg od

Increase to max dose of 400 mg/day (in divided doses)
Diuresis can take up to 5 days to have full effect
Stop if Na+ < 120 mmol/L

Formulary (continued)

Drug	Preparations	Indications	Dose
Sucralfate	Tablet: 1 g Suspension: 1 g/5 mL	Duodenal or gastric ulcer Chronic gastritis Surface bleeding	Duodenal or gastric ulcer and chronic gastritis: 2 g bd or 1 g qds Surface bleeding: 1–2 g
Tapentadol	Normal release: 50 and 75 mg Modified release: 50, 100, 150, 200 and 250 mg	Moderate to severe pain	Initially 50 mg every 4–6 hours Max. 600 mg daily or with modified release 50 mg every 12 hours Max dose 500 mg daily
Temazepam	Tablet: 10 or 20 mg Oral solution: 10 mg/5 mL	Insomnia	10–20 mg in the evening
Thalidomide		Cachexia Sweating	Cachexia: 100–200 mg in the evening Sweating: 100–200 mg in the evening
Tramadol	Capsule: 50 mg Orodispersible tablet: 50 mg Injection: 50 mg/mL	Moderate-to-severe pain	50–100 mg qds Max dose 400 mg/day
Tranexamic acid	Tablet: 500 mg	Capillary bleeding	Orally: 1–1.5 g bd/qds Topical : 0.5–1 g directly on to wound
Venlafaxine	Tablet: 37.5 or 75 mg	Antidepressant Anxiety Neuropathic pain Hot flushes	37.5–75 mg bd
Zoledronic acid	Concentrate for intravenous infusion: 4 mg/5 mL	Bone pain Hypercalcemia	4–8 mg every 4–6 weeks
Zolpidem	Tablet: 5 or 10 mg	Insomnia	5 mg in the evening
Zopiclone	Tablet: 3.75 or 7.5 mg	Insomnia	3.75 mg in the evening

Figure A.3.1 Formulary (continued). *Bd* twice daily, *CNS* central nervous system, *CSCI* continuous subcutaneous infusion, *EC* enteric coated, *GABA* γ-aminobutyric acid, *GI* gastrointestinal, *h* hour, *HT* hydroxytryptamine (serotonin), *im* intramuscularly, *iv* intravenously, *max* maximum, *NSAID* non-steroidal anti-inflammatory drug, *od* once daily, *PHN* post-herpetic neuralgia, *po* orally, *PPI* proton pump inhibitor, *prn* as required, *q3h* 3 hourly, *q4h* 4 hourly, *q6h* 6 hourly, *q8h* 8 hourly, *qds* four times daily, *sc* subcutaneously, *SCC* spinal cord compression, *sl* sublingually, *SNRI* serotonin–norepinephrine reuptake inhibitor, *SVCO* superior vena cava obstruction, *stat* immediately, *TD* transdermal, *tds* three times daily

Notes

Should be taken for 4–6 weeks. Dose can be increased to max 8 g/day
Suspension (for oral lesions) or crushed tablet (in Intrasite gel) can be used for surface bleeding

Tapentadol is a new molecule that has both opioid and non-opioid activity

Can be increased to 30–40 mg as necesssary
Usually reserved for short-term use

Capsule must be swallowed whole

12-hour modified-release formulation available (50, 100, 150, or 200 mg)
24-hour modified-release formulation available (100, 150, 200, 300 or 400 mg)
Combination with paracetamol/acetaminophen (Tramacet: tramadol 37.5 mg + paracetamol 325 mg)

For oral use consider reducing dose after 7 days once bleeding has stopped.
For topical application use injection or crushed tablets and review after 20 minutes

SNRI; modified-release formulations available (75, 150, or 225 mg)
Increase as necessary to 75 mg bd. With specialits advice can be increased further in75-mg steps every 2–3 days to max dose 375 mg
For anxiety 75 mg modified release od. If no response after 8 weeks discontinue

Inhibitor of osteoclastic bone resorption
Max response for hypercalcemia seen after 4 days
Relief for bone pain can take up to 14 days
Osteonecrosis of the jaw a potential complication

Can be increased to 10 mg in the evening if necessary
Can be increased to 7.5 mg if required

Step 2 combination preparations and daily morphine equivalent	
Preparation	**Constituents**
Co-codamol 8/500	Codeine + paracetamol/acetaminophen
Co-codaprin 8/400	Codeine + aspirin
Co-codamol 15/500	Codeine + paracetamol/acetaminophen
Co-codamol 30/500	Codeine + paracetamol/acetaminophen
Co-dydramol 10/500	Dihydrocodeine + paracetamol/acetaminophen
Remedeine 20/500	Dihydrocodeine + paracetamol/acetaminophen
Remedeine Forte 30/500	Dihydrocodeine + paracetamol/acetaminophen

Figure A.3.2 **Step 2 combination preparations and daily morphine equivalent.** *Tabs* tablets

Approximate hypnotics – equivalent dose of benzodiazepines	
Diazepam	5 mg
Chlordiazepoxide	15 mg
Loprazolam	0.5–1.0 mg
Lorazepam	500 µg
Lormetazepam	0.5–1.0 mg
Nitrazepam	5 mg
Oxazepam	15 mg
Temazepam	10 mg

Figure A.3.3 **Approximate hypnotics – equivalent dose of benzodiazepines**

Dose	Max daily dose (mg)	Daily morphine equivalence (mg)
1–2 tabs 4–6 hours	8	6.4
1–2 tabs 4–6 hours	8	6.4
1–2 tabs 4–6 hours	8	12
1–2 tabs 4–6 hours	8	24
1–2 tabs 4–6 hours	8	10
1–2 tabs 4–6 hours	8	20
1–2 tabs 4–6 hours	8	30

Equivalent anti-inflammatory doses of corticosteroids	
Prednisolone	5 mg
Betamethasone	750 µg
Cortisone acetate	25 mg
Deflazacort	6 mg
Dexamethasone	750 µg
Hydrocortisone	20 mg
Methylprednisolone	4 mg
Triamcinolone	4 mg

Figure A.3.4 Equivalent anti-inflammatory doses of corticosteroids

References

1. Zigmond AS, Snaith RP. The hospital anxiety and depression scale. Acta Psychiatr Scand. 1983;67:361–70.
2. Jacobsen PB, Donovan KA, Trask PC, et al. Screening for psychological distress in ambulatory cancer patients. Cancer. 2005;103:1494–502.
3. Hodkinson HM. Evaluation of a mental test score for assessment of mental impairment in the elderly. Age Ageing. 1972;1:233–8.
4. Cleeland CS, Ryan KM. Pain assessment: global use of the Brief Pain Inventory. Ann Acad Med Singapore. 1994;23:129–38.
5. Bennett M. The LANSS pain scale: the Leeds assessment of neuropathic symptoms and signs. Pain. 2001;92:147–57.
6. Netter F. Dermatome map of the body. Atlas of human anatomy. 5th ed. Philadelphia: Saunders; 2010. p. 159.
7. Zeppetella G, Ribeiro MD. Episodic pain in patients with advanced cancer. Am J Hosp Palliat Care. 2002;19:267–76.

Index

G. Zeppetella, *Palliative Care in Clinical Practice*,
DOI 10.1007/978-1-4471-2843-4,
© Springer-Verlag London 2012

Printed by Printforce, the Netherlands